YOUR BODY. YOUR HEALTH.
YOUR IDEAL SUPPLEMENT PLAN
IN 3 EASY STEPS

No two people are alike. And when it comes to supplements, everyone's needs are different. This unique book recognizes that choosing the right herbs, vitamins, and minerals for your body is crucial to achieving optimum health. And with the dynamic step-by-step program outlined here, you'll get all the essential information you need to design a supplement plan that's tailor-made for you.

Are you concerned about cholesterol? Battling insomnia? Do you want to boost your immune system? Reduce stress? Alleviate symptoms of the flu? Whatever your individual health concerns, this authoritative reference helps you to choose the perfect supplements for you . . . providing invaluable information on dosages, drug interactions, side effects, and much, much more.

YOUR IDEAL SUPPLEMENT PLAN IN 3 EASY STEPS

The Essential Guide to Choosing the Herbs, Vitamins, and Minerals That Are Right for You

DEBORAH MITCHELL

foreword by Hunter Yost, M.D.

A LYNN SONBERG BOOK
A DELL BOOK

Published by
Dell Publishing
a division of
Random House, Inc.
1540 Broadway
New York, New York 10036

IMPORTANT NOTE:

This book is for informational purposes only. It is not intended to take the place of medical advice from a trained medical professional. Readers are advised to consult a physician or other qualified health professional regarding treatment of all of their health problems or before acting on any of the information or advice in this book.

This book is intended to provide selected information about vitamins, minerals, herbal remedies, and other supplements. Research about herbal medicine is ongoing and subject to conflicting interpretations. As a result, there is no guarantee that what we know about this subject won't change with time.

Cover photo copyright © 2000 by Shaun Egan / Tony Stone Images
Cover design by Melody Cassen
Book design by Ellen Cipriano
Copyright © 2000 by Lynn Sonberg Book Associates

Dell books may be purchased for business or promotional use or for special sales. For information please write to: Special Markets Department, Random House, Inc., 1540 Broadway, New York, N.Y. 10036.

Dell® is a registered trademark of Random House, Inc., and the colophon is a trademark of Random House, Inc.

ISBN: 0-440-23554-5

Published by arrangement with
Lynn Sonberg Book Associates
10 West 86 Street
New York, N.Y. 10024
Printed in the United States of America
Published simultaneously in Canada

January 2000

10 9 8 7 6 5 4 3 2 1

OPM

CONTENTS

PART II: COMMON MEDICAL CONDITIONS AND AILMENTS

PART III: YOUR OPTIMAL SUPPLEMENT PROGRAM

Foreword

❧

The father of medicine, Hippocrates, once said, "A wise man should consider that health is the greatest of human blessings." We all know this to be true, in our heart of hearts, yet how many of us are truly wise when it comes to our health? More specifically, how many people eat the kind of diet that promotes and supports health and well-being? The sad truth is, not many. How many people eat five or more servings of fruits and vegetables a day? Only about ten percent of people follow this advice from the American Institute for Cancer Research, the World Cancer Research Fund, and many other health organizations. Even a smaller percentage eat only whole, organic foods, or avoid food additives, caffeine, sugar, and alcohol. And how many people frequent fa(s)t-food burger restaurants? It's no wonder so many people are tired, sick, and overweight.

Yet while many people are striving to do more in their lives, they're also giving themselves less to do it on. If you do not fuel your body well and consistently, you'll run at half throttle and place undue stress on all your organs and body functions. When that happens, you are highly susceptible to infection and disease. The link between stress and illness is undeniable. But knowing that you should do something and then actually doing it are two different things. And you do want to feel better and be healthier, or you wouldn't have picked up this book. Congratulations; that's the "should" side of the equation. *Your Ideal Supplement Plan in 3 Easy Steps* shows you the "doing" side. It explains how you can take an active part in attaining, restoring, and maintaining your health with a supplement plan that is designed especially for you, by you. And it doesn't have to be hard. In fact, you can do it in three steps.

A supplement plan that addresses your particular needs can be one of the most important things you do for your health. In my practice, I see many people get dramatic results once nutritional deficiencies have been corrected or they have decided to take natural remedies for conditions such as arthritis, allergies, chronic fatigue, and headache. That is not to say that conventional treatments should be ignored or discarded. In fact, natural approaches can complement them when they are needed. The truth is, however, that in many cases conventional medicine is not necessary. Natural remedies work with the body instead of against it, allowing it to draw upon its inherent healing powers. Taking natural supplements also gives individuals a sense of control over their own bodies and their own health. This sense of being in charge is an integral part of the healing process.

Yet even though the rewards of good health are priceless, many people do not do it. Two of the most common reasons people give for not taking better care of their health are "I'm too busy" and "It's too confusing because there are so many supplements." *Your Ideal Supplement Plan in 3 Easy Steps* addresses both of these concerns.

"I'm too busy." It is so characteristic of our society to wait until something is wrong with our health before we do anything about it. We barrel along in life, believing (and hoping) that we won't get sick, that it happens only to the "other guy." But many diseases and ailments can be avoided or their effects greatly reduced if we take just a minute or two a day to give the body what it needs. It's a minute well spent, especially when you compare it with the days, weeks, months, or even years you can be sick if you stop paying attention to your body and its nutritional requirements.

Fortunately, this type of preventive medicine is catching on. People are beginning to realize that a one- or two-minute investment each day yields excellent returns, often noticeable almost immediately. Taking supplements may not solve all your health problems, but depending on your individual needs, it can enhance and maintain your current health, restore faltering health, or put you on a new road to well-being. Even if you have a chronic condition such as diabetes or multiple sclerosis, natural remedies can significantly improve your quality of life by promoting natural healing processes.

"It's too confusing," and that is true. Walk into any nutrition store or pharmacy and the supplement displays can be overwhelming. But this book helps take away the confusion and replaces it with a practical, easy-to-follow way to choose the supplements that are best for you, whether you want only to enhance your vitality, you need to treat an acute condition such as headache or diarrhea, or you have a more persistent condition, such as irritable bowel syndrome or gingivitis. If you have questions about the supplements that are not answered here, or if you are taking medications or have a serious medical condition, you may want to consult with a health-care professional who is knowledgeable about nutrition before starting a supplement program. And you can take this book with you, because it offers basic, concise, and comprehensive information on more than seventy supplements and more than sixty medical conditions and ailments. All it takes is three easy-to-follow steps and you can be on your way to better health and more energy.

HUNTER YOST, M.D.

YOUR INTRODUCTION TO
SUPPLEMENTATION

Walk into your neighborhood pharmacy, drugstore, nutrition or health-food store, and chances are you are bombarded with a dizzying number of supplement choices. Even many supermarkets now have shelf after shelf of vitamins, minerals, herbal formulas, and other nutritional supplements for sale. From vitamin A to zinc, amino acids to wild yam, acidophilus to yohimbé, the bottles taunt you, vying for your attention and your dollars. Before you walked into the store you thought you knew what you wanted and needed; now you feel overwhelmed and as if you need a PhD to figure out what to buy.

This book takes the confusion out of choosing the supplements that are the most beneficial for you. It gives you detailed, useful information about the most helpful and common health-enhancing supplements in several key categories: vitamins and minerals, herbal remedies, and a group of miscellaneous supplements too diverse to fit into a neat category: a few enzymes, amino acids, oils, hormones, phytochemicals (chemicals from plants), and other gifts from nature. It then shows you how you can take this wealth of information and customize a supplement program that fits your unique needs and lifestyle, including taking into account any specific diseases or medical conditions you may have, be they long- or short-term, temporary or chronic. *Your Ideal Supplement Plan in 3 Easy Steps* answers the questions that cross the mind of nearly every supplement consumer, questions about why supplements are important, which forms are best to take, differences between natural and synthetic supplements, where to buy supplements, and questions about terms on supplement packaging, such as *antioxidant, chelated, standardized, USP*—terms that can be daunting when you're standing in the supplement aisle. (These terms are discussed under "Shop for Your Health-Enhancing Supplements" within Part III of the book.) First, however, you need to consider the big question.

Do I Need to Take Supplements?

You've heard it time and time again, from doctors and in news reports, in articles on nutrition and in countless books: good nutrition is an essential foundation for good health. But good nutrition is about more than just making sure you get enough of a few vitamins and minerals: more than forty nutrients are required by the body to help it keep functioning properly. Of those nutrients the Council for Responsible Nutrition reports that most Americans are deficient in many, including vitamins A, C, E, thiamin, riboflavin, B_6, B_{12}, and folic acid, and the nutrients calcium, chromium, iron, magnesium, selenium, and zinc.

But good health is about more than vitamins and minerals. Scientific investigations into the medicinal value of herbs, phytochemicals, enzymes, hormones, and other natural supplements have led researchers and physicians to appreciate the health-enhancing properties of these compounds. Although the research into these supplements is not as extensive as that of most vitamins and minerals, it is being pursued vigorously by investigators around the world, providing the general public with more and more natural, safe choices when it comes to healthy supplements.

Although most people know that eating whole, natural foods and drinking pure water are crucial elements in a healthy diet, many continue to follow the Standard American Diet—SAD—which, true to its acronym, is sadly deficient in nutrients and fiber and high in fat, cholesterol, and toxins. Even if you include many fresh fruits, vegetables, and whole grains in your diet, conventionally grown foods are usually raised in nutritionally deficient soil and thus are lacking in nutrients themselves. The trip from the field to your table, which includes processing, transporting, storing, and cooking, can destroy many of the remaining nutrients. Eating organically grown fruits, vegetables, and grains and avoiding processed foods is one way to help ensure you are getting the nutrients your body needs.

Other factors that can also hinder your body from getting the proper nutritional value from your food include stress, environmental pollutants, and medical conditions. Emotional and physical stress can cause a breakdown of your immune system and make you susceptible to invasion by harmful microorganisms and result in countless problems, from the common cold to ulcers to heart disease, all of which can hinder how your body absorbs or uses nutrients. Stress also increases your body's requirements for many nutrients, especially the water-soluble vitamins such as vitamin C and the B vitamins. That's why, for example, you can buy vitamin combinations sold as "stress formulas," which contain the B vitamins and often vitamin C as well.

Environmental pollutants, such as cigarette smoke and gasoline fumes, can promote the formation of harmful substances known as free radicals (see "Antioxidant" question in Part III), which also can alter how your body absorbs and uses food. Medical conditions can have varying effects on how your food is processed: for example, diarrhea causes the body to lose vital nutrients and fluids rapidly, while many people with irritable bowel syndrome are sensitive to foods such as wheat and so must be careful about the foods they eat.

These factors, and many more, lead to the need for supplements. Many physicians, nutritionists, and researchers agree that everyone needs to take supplemental nutrients, even if only a multivitamin-mineral combination, because no one escapes the one factor that causes changes in how the body absorbs and utilizes nutrients—aging. As we grow older, the body loses some of its ability to assimilate the nutrients we take in. In addition, the levels of many important nutrients—for example, the amino acids methionine and cysteine; many of the antioxidants, such as coenzyme Q10 and vitamin E; and DHEA, which is a precursor for many hormones—decline with age. Supplementation, while it cannot stop aging, can help make the trip smoother and healthier.

Supplements are an insurance policy against such unknowns as What is the true nutritional value of the food I eat? How many toxins are in my food? What effect are emotional and physical stress having on my body's ability to utilize nutrients?

Health-enhancing supplements can both help you maintain health and help restore it when you develop a medical condition or disease. A problem for many people is knowing which supplements are best for them—for helping them maintain good health and for when they have a specific condition they wish to treat. This book can help you make those decisions, easily and with confidence.

How to Use This Book

Too often, people get home with supplements in hand and then don't know how best to take them. They've "heard" or "read" about specific herbs or nutritional supplements that help relieve headache or arthritis or that help prevent cancer, but don't really know what to do with the supplements once they get them home. Here's where *Your Ideal Supplement Plan in 3 Easy Steps* can help. The book is divided into three easy-to-follow parts. Part I contains an alphabetical list of more than sixty health-enhancing supplements and the details you need to buy and use them; information such as:

- What are the best forms to buy?
- What dosage should I take?
- How many times a day should I take it?
- Should I take the supplement with food or on an empty stomach?
- Are there foods or drugs I should avoid when taking certain supplements?
- Are there specific supplements I should take together in order to increase their beneficial actions?
- Are the supplements safe to take if I have a specific medical condition or if I'm pregnant?

Each supplement entry also includes, in **bold** type, the medical conditions and diseases that can be treated with the supplement. Each **bold** word or phrase can be found in Part II, where dozens of ailments are explained and the most appropriate supplements to treat them are listed, along with the suggested dosage.

Part III gives you the tools to create your own ideal supplement program. First, it offers you a summary of the information in Parts I and II in an easy-to-read chart. Then it presents the three simple steps to build a health-enhancing program tailored for you and provides you with the building blocks you need. If you encounter a term that is unfamiliar to you, refer to the Glossary that follows Part III.

It's that easy. Now welcome to the world of better health through supplementation.

PART I

SUPPLEMENTS: NATURE'S INSURANCE POLICIES

Supplements can be the best insurance policy you ever buy. They give you the power to attain and maintain the most precious thing you can ever possess—your health. Just as important as having the physical supplements in your possession and taking them are the emotional, mental, and spiritual benefits you experience from knowing you are taking an active part in creating balance and health for yourself.

In the Introduction you learned some basic things about supplements and why you need them. In this section you can learn about the most commonly used supplements and how they are helpful, what forms to buy, how to use them, what side effects and interactions to look for, foods that contain the nutrient (if applicable), signs of deficiency (if applicable), and precautions.

A Note about "What to Buy": The majority of supplements are available in more than one form; some in as many as eight or ten. Not all forms are equally effective, which is why "What to Buy" lets you know which ones are more beneficial. In addition, where applicable it lists

"Other Helpful Supplements" forms for those who cannot obtain readily the recommended forms in their area or who prefer to take the alternative forms.

When purchasing supplements sight unseen via mail order or the Internet, get as much information about the products as you can by calling the company's customer service department. Comparison-shop: check out several suppliers; look for advertisements in health and nutrition publications; ask your physician, pharmacist, and knowledgeable staff in health-food stores. Read labels carefully and research the options. Sometimes a store brand may serve your needs just as well as a higher-priced national label.

An explanation of several terms you will see often in this section will be helpful. *Standardized* and *standardized extract* are used to describe many herbal supplements. *Standardized* means that the herb form is guaranteed to contain a predetermined, or standardized, level of active ingredients. A standardized extract can be a solid, liquid, or powder. Any form of an herb can be standardized; however, not all manufacturers have adopted this practice. Whenever possible, buy the standardized form of the herb(s) you have chosen to take, as it is the preferred and more effective form of an herb.

Some herbs can be taken as an "infusion" or a "decoction." Both forms are prepared similarly to teas, with two important differences: in both cases more herb is used than in ordinary tea; and the herb is allowed to steep longer. These differences make infusions and decoctions much more potent than average tea. Infusions are prepared from the soft parts of the herb—leaves, flowers, and berries. Decoctions are made from the hard parts—bark, roots, and stems.

A Note about "How to Use": The doses provided in the "How to Use" section are a general guide. Because there are many different manufacturers of supplement products and various potencies, it is necessary to read the dosing directions on each product before you use it. For more detailed dosing information, refer to the specific condition (in **bold** type) you are treating. Check the package instructions and consult with your health-care provider before taking any supplement.

The dosage instructions have been drawn from a wide variety of authoritative sources, including highly regarded medical practitioners and institutions. For a complete list of sources, see page 228. Doses are given in milligrams (mg, or thousandths of a gram); micrograms (mcg, or millionths of a gram); and milliliters (mL, or thousandths of a liter). See Appendix C for measurement conversions.

ACIDOPHILUS Acidophilus (*Lactobacillus acidophilus*) is a type of beneficial bacteria that resides in the colon and vagina. Acidophilus helps destroy bad bacteria, promotes the growth of good bacteria, improves digestion, and boosts the immune system. One common use of acidophilus is in the prevention and treatment of yeast infections (see vaginitis), which can inhabit the intestines as well as other organs in the body. Acidophilus is also used to treat and prevent **athlete's foot, canker sores, chronic fatigue syndrome, diarrhea, diverticulitus, fibrocystic breast disease, herpes, inflammatory bowel disease, irritable bowel syndrome, multiple sclerosis,** and **urinary-tract infections.**

Acidophilus is the main beneficial bacteria in the small intestine, where it replenishes the colonies of good bacteria. Regular supplementation with acidophilus can help maintain a healthy balance of beneficial bacteria and thus inhibit the growth of harmful microorganisms, especially among women who are susceptible to yeast infections. Individuals who are especially likely to be deficient in good bacteria are those taking antibiotics or eating a poor diet, or anyone experiencing diarrhea, especially chronic cases. Active live cultures of acidophilus are found in some brands of yogurt and in acidophilus milk, but the concentration of acidophilus is higher in the supplement.

What to Buy: Powder and liquid extracts are preferred. Acidophilus is available with either a dairy (cow or goat milk) or nondairy (carrot juice, apple pectin) base. The nondairy form is recommended, especially if you are or suspect you may be lactose intolerant. Although acidophilus is also sold as a combination product containing more than one strain of lactobacilli, most experts recommend using a single-strain product. Look for brands that tell you specifically how many CFUs (colony-forming units) you get per dose (see "How to Use"). Do not buy any product that uses the preservative BHT.

Also available as a capsule, tablet (chewable), and softgel.

How to Use: The recommended daily dose depends on whether you are treating a condition, such as a yeast infection, or whether you are using it for preventive purposes. Acidophilus should be taken on an empty stomach and one hour before meals. The typical dosage is 1 to 2 billion CFUs per day, which generally means any one of the following forms three times a day: 2 Tbs powder in cool liquid (not hot); or 1 Tbs liquid extract. See individual medical entries for specific dosages.

Possible Side Effects and Precautions: No side effects have been reported. People who have an intestinal disorder should consult their physician before taking acidophilus. Because heat can kill acidophilus, store the supplement in the refrigerator, and do not take it in hot or warm liquids.

Be aware of the expiration date on the bottle, because the bacteria must be alive to be beneficial.

Interactions: Use of acidophilus may help promote production of folic acid, biotin, vitamin B_6, and niacin.

ALFALFA The dried leaves of alfalfa (*Medicago sativa*) have been used for centuries to treat various disorders of the gastrointestinal tract, including loss of appetite and indigestion. It is still used for these conditions, as well as for high cholesterol, **flatulence, irritable bowel syndrome,** and **nausea.** Some controversy, however, surrounds the use of alfalfa (see "Precautions" below).

Alfalfa leaves contain saponins, which appear to prevent absorption of cholesterol. Other substances in the leaves include chlorophyll, flavones, isoflavones, sterols, protein, calcium, magnesium, potassium, and all known vitamins. Overall, alfalfa leaves are thought to cleanse the body by acting as a laxative and diuretic and by stimulating the appetite.

What to Buy: Tincture, powdered extracts, and capsules are recommended. Also available as dried leaves. The infusions made from dried leaves generally do not deliver enough active ingredients to be effective.

How to Take: No therapeutic dose of alfalfa has been identified, but some experts recommend taking 1 to 2 mL tincture daily. Powdered extract and capsules should be taken according to package directions. See individual medical conditions for specific dosages.

Possible Side Effects and Precautions: Diarrhea and stomach upset occur occasionally. Stop taking the supplement immediately and consult your health-care provider. People with lupus or a history of the disease should avoid all alfalfa products. People with anemia should take alfalfa only with the permission of their physician, as the saponins in alfalfa can damage red blood cells.

Interactions: If combining alfalfa with other herbs, you may need to reduce the dosage of alfalfa.

ALOE VERA Of the more than 120 types of aloe the one most commonly grown and used is the aloe vera (*Aloe vera*). The healing powers of aloe vera lie in its fleshy leaves, which contain a sticky gel and latex. The gel contains polysaccharides, which make it an effective external treatment for burns, cuts, **acne, shingles,** and other skin irritations. Latex, which is taken orally, is a bitter yellow liquid that treats **constipation, heartburn, irritable bowel syndrome,** gastritis, and stomach **ulcers.** Aloe vera contains anthraquinones, substances that can reduce the growth of calcium crystals that cause **kidney stones.** Some experts also believe aloe vera can eliminate kidney stones once they form.

What to Buy: Recommended forms are the bottled gel (juice), latex tablets, fluid extract, and lotion (for external use). Also available as powder, powdered capsules, and softgels.

How to Use: The gel, latex tablets, and softgels are often used for **constipation** (see entry for dosage). Any other internal use of aloe, including taking the gel for **ulcers, diverticulitis,** and other gastrointestinal problems, should be done under the guidance of a physician. The powder and powdered capsules can also be taken for gastrointestinal disorders. Topical use of the gel is effective for skin problems. See individual medical entries for specific dosages.

Possible Side Effects and Precautions: Rash, diarrhea, or intestinal cramps are possible. Reduce the dose or stop taking the supplement. If you have a gastrointestinal condition, do not take aloe without first consulting your physician. Pregnant or lactating women can use aloe externally but should avoid using it internally. Do not exceed the recommended dose of aloe latex.

Interactions: If you combine aloe with other herbs, you may need to reduce the dose.

ASTRAGALUS More than two thousand types of astragalus are found around the world, but the species most studied is the Chinese version, huang qi. Astragalus (*Astragalus membranaceus*), also known as milk vetch, contains polysaccharides, which experts believe are responsible for its healing abilities. This perennial herb is used to treat chronic **cancer, chronic fatigue,** and **colds and flu.** Its effectiveness against these immune-system conditions may be at least partially attributed to the high level of the antioxidant selenium in astragalus.

The Chinese use astragalus in fu-zheng therapy, the treatment of conditions in which the body's immune system needs to be strengthened. Of particular interest is its use in cancer patients undergoing radiation and/or chemotherapy. Some Western investigators believe this herb may be somewhat effective in this role. Researchers at M. D. Anderson Hospital in Houston, Texas, for example, concluded that astragalus protects the liver from the adverse effects of chemotherapy and that it can restore T-cell function to normal.

What to Buy: Recommended are the tincture and extract. Also available as capsules containing dried root and prepared tea bags.

How to Use: Tincture and extract—3 to 5 mL ($^1/_8$ to $^1/_2$ tsp) three times daily. Dried root capsules—250 to 500 mg two to three times daily with meals or water. Prepare the tea bag according to package directions. See individual medical entries for specific dosages.

Possible Side Effects and Precautions: No side effects noted. If you are pregnant, check with your doctor before taking astragalus.

BEE POLLEN Many experts believe bee pollen is one of the richest natural sources of vitamins, minerals, amino acids, protein (10 to 35 percent), and other nutrients. Bee pollen is harvested from beehives that are specifically modified to collect flower pollen as it falls from the bees' legs. The pollen is used to boost energy and endurance levels, treat **prostate problems** and **sinusitis,** and reduce stress and fatigue. Some experts claim bee pollen can also be effective in treating arthritis, cancer, heart conditions, and intestinal problems, although none of these claims have been proven scientifically.

What to Buy: Recommended forms are capsules and tablets, 100 to 500 mg each, and liquid.

How to Use: Tablets and capsules—250 to 1,500 mg daily. Because some people (fewer than 1 percent) are allergic to bee pollen, take one-half tablet or capsule to see if you get an allergic reaction, such as rash or wheezing. Gradually increase the dose over a few days to ensure you are not allergic to the supplement. Take liquid according to package directions. See individual medical entries for specific dosages.

Possible Side Effects: Mild, transient side effects include rash, itching, and swelling. Serious effects include anaphylactic shock, characterized by severe itching, drop in blood pressure, swelling, loss of breath, and loss of consciousness.

Precautions: Do not take bee pollen if you are allergic to bee stings, if you have kidney disease or gout, or if you are pregnant or breast-feeding. Bee pollen is not the same as flower pollen, which is also sold as a supplement. If you are allergic to airborne pollen, you may have a negative reaction to bee pollen.

BILBERRY The bilberry (*Vaccinium myrtillus*), a relative of the blueberry, grows in the United States, Europe, and Canada. Its dried berries and leaves are used to treat **cata-**

racts, glaucoma, macular degeneration, vomiting, and **varicose veins.** Bilberry helps prevent or heal fragile capillaries and other small blood vessels, which improves blood flow. These benefits appear to come from chemicals in the berries called anthocyanosides, which reportedly are up to fifty times more potent than vitamin E in antioxidant power.

What to Buy: Standardized forms are preferred—capsules, tincture, or fluid extract standardized to provide 25 percent anthocyanosides. Also available as dried leaves and dried berries.

How to Use: General dosages include 240 to 480 mg daily of standardized capsules; 80 to 160 mg daily of standardized fluid extract. To prepare an infusion, boil 2 to 3 tsp dried leaves in 1 cup water. Take 1 cup per day. For dried berries, simmer 1 cup water and 1 tsp dried berries for fifteen minutes. Drink 1 to 2 cups per day, cold. See individual medical entries for specific dosages.

Possible Side Effects and Precautions: No side effects noted when taken as directed. Do not eat fresh bilberries, as they can cause diarrhea.

Interactions: Bilberry does not interact with prescription drugs.

BIOTIN Biotin is a member of the water-soluble B vitamin family. Also known as B_7 and vitamin H, biotin is found in soy, whole grains, egg yolk, almonds, walnuts, oatmeal, mushrooms, broccoli, bananas, peanuts, and nutritional yeast. Its primary functions in the body are to assist with the metabolism of fats, carbohydrates, and proteins; help with cell growth; and facilitate the utilization of the other B vitamins.

Biotin has proved helpful in lowering and controlling the blood sugar levels in people with either insulin-dependent or noninsulin-dependent **diabetes. Seborrheic der-**

matitis, a common skin disorder among infants and adults, is believed to be caused by a biotin deficiency among infants, while biotin's role among adults with this condition is not certain.

A deficiency of biotin can cause depression, hair loss, high blood sugar, anemia, loss of appetite, insomnia, muscular pain, nausea, and a sore tongue. Biotin deficiency is very rare, because this vitamin can be manufactured by the intestines from other foods. Long-term use of antibiotics, however, can hinder production of biotin and lead to deficiency symptoms. Signs of deficiency are also seen in people who regularly consume raw egg whites, which contain a protein called avidin that prevents absorption of biotin.

What to Buy: Purchase either a multivitamin-mineral supplement or a B-complex formula that contains biotin. Most people do not need to take a separate biotin supplement unless they are treating **diabetes,** in which case it is recommended you do so under a doctor's guidance.

How to Use: **Note: These dosages are for adults only. Consult with your physician before giving biotin to an infant.** No dietary reference intake has been established for biotin. Not all physicians agree as to the recommended daily dose. Some say 30 to 100 mcg is adequate for maintenance of health; others suggest 300 mcg. For people with diabetes, intake may be as high as 8 to 16 mg per day.

Possible Side Effects and Precautions: Biotin is a water-soluble vitamin; thus, if excessive amounts are taken, they are excreted in the urine without causing adverse effects. People with diabetes who are taking insulin will need to decrease their insulin dosage if they take more than 8 mg biotin daily.

Interactions: Biotin works in conjunction with the other B vitamins. Substances that can interfere with bioavailability of biotin include antibiotics, saccharin, and sulfa drugs.

BLACK COHOSH Black cohosh (*Cimicifuga racemosa*) is a leafy, shrublike perennial that has been used for centuries to relieve **menopause-** and **PMS-**related pain and discomfort (especially hot flashes), and **endometriosis.** Its healing power lies in its roots and rhizome, which contain an estrogenlike substance called formononetin. Formononetin helps reduce the secretion of luteinizing hormone, which is responsible for hot flashes and other menopausal symptoms. Black cohosh also has sedative abilities.

What to Buy: The standardized extract, powdered extract, and tincture are preferred. Also available as dried root or rhizome, capsules, syrup.

How to Use: Powdered extract—250 mg three times per day in water or juice. Tincture—2 to 4 mL per day. Standardized extract—40 mg twice daily. Capsules—two 20 mg daily. To prepare a decoction from the dried root or rhizome, add 1/2 tsp to 1 cup boiling water. Cover and let steep and cool for thirty minutes. Take 2 Tbs at a time as needed, up to 1 cup per day, cold. Do not take black cohosh for longer than six months. See individual medical entries for specific dosages.

Possible Side Effects: Contact your physician if you experience any of these side effects: irritated uterus, nausea, headache, drop in blood pressure and/or heart rate, diarrhea, stomach pain, joint pain, breast tumors, blood clots.

Precautions: Because serious side effects are possible, this herb should be taken under medical supervision. Do not take black cohosh if you are pregnant, have heart disease, are taking estrogen therapy, are lactating, or if you have been advised not to take oral contraceptives.

Interactions: No interactions have been reported.

BORON Boron is a trace mineral that plays an important role in the metabolism of calcium, magnesium, and phosphorus; the enhancement of brain functioning; maintenance of strong bones; and the promotion of mental alertness. Boron appears to help prevent **osteoporosis** in postmenopausal women by increasing the absorption of calcium and phosphorus. It is also used to relieve the symptoms of **osteoarthritis** and **backache.** No cases of boron deficiency have been reported. Foods that contain boron include raisins, almonds, prunes, and most fruits (except citrus) and leafy vegetables.

What to Buy: Look for a multivitamin-mineral supplement that contains boron. Also suggested are tablets or powder. Regardless of the form you choose, look for either boron citrate or boron aspartate, or a combination of the two, plus glycinate chelates.

How to Use: Experts recommend taking 1 to 3 mg per day, with food. The elderly need 2 to 3 mg daily, because their ability to absorb calcium is reduced. See individual medical entries for specific dosages.

Possible Side Effects and Precautions: No adverse effects have been noted when boron is taken at recommended levels. At a dosage of more than 3 mg per day, estrogen levels may rise, which can increase the risk of cancer.

Interactions: Boron may help the body conserve its supply of calcium, magnesium, and phosphorus.

BOSWELLIA Also known as guggal, boswellia (*Boswellia serrata*) is a tree that grows in India. A gummy oleoresin, also called guggal, is found in the tree trunk and consists of boswellic acids, which have antiinflammatory properties. Boswellia has been a favorite antiarthritic therapy among Ayurvedic practitioners for centuries. Today it is used to treat **osteoarthritis, rheumatoid arthritis, bursitis,** and ulcerative colitis, as well as bronchoconstrictive conditions such as asthma.

What to Buy: The standardized extract containing 37.5 to 65 percent boswellic acids is preferred. For topical use, buy the cream in a base of *Boswellia serrata* and standardized for boswellic acids. Some creams also contain vitamin E. Boswellia is also available as tablets.

How to Use: Extract—400 mg three times daily if standardized to 37.5 percent; 200 mg three times daily if standardized to 65 percent. Cream is for external use only. See individual medical entries for specific dosages.

Possible Side Effects and Precautions: Rare; can include diarrhea, rash, and nausea. Avoid using if pregnant or lactating.

BREWER'S YEAST Yeast is a single-celled organism that multiplies rapidly and is rich in many nutrients, including sixteen amino acids, all the B vitamins except B_{12} (some forms do contain B_{12}), at least fourteen minerals, and seventeen vitamins. Brewer's yeast can be grown from several different sources: from hops, when it's known as nutritional yeast; or from blackstrap molasses or wood pulp, which produces tourla yeast. Brewer's yeast differs from baker's yeast in that the latter has live yeast cells that deplete the body of B vitamins and other nutrients. These live cells are eliminated in brewer's yeast.

Conditions that often respond to supplementation with brewer's yeast include fatigue, skin irritations, nervousness, **diabetes,** and **diarrhea.** Brewer's yeast also reportedly improves mental effectiveness and boosts the immune system.

What to Buy: Look for high-quality brands that contain about 60 mcg chromium per tablespoon (or flakes or powder) or tablet. Only true brewer's yeast has chromium.

How to Use: Flakes and powder can be added to food or beverages. Mix in $^{1}/_{2}$ to 2 Tbs two to three times daily.

Brewer's yeast has a cheesy taste, thus sprinkling it on cooked vegetables, mashed potatoes, or pasta makes it easy and enjoyable to take. Tablets—1 three times daily. See individual medical entries for specific dosages.

Possible Side Effects and Precautions: None reported.

BROMELAIN Bromelain is a mixture of protein-digesting enzymes found in pineapple. It inhibits the action of proinflammatory substances and prevents the production of kinins, compounds produced during the inflammatory process that cause pain. Research shows that it also promotes circulation, reduces the stickiness of platelets in the blood, reduces bruising, and aids in digestion.

Bromelain is an effective antiinflammatory agent for treatment of **carpal tunnel syndrome, bursitis, sinusitis, varicose veins,** sports injuries, menstrual cramps, and postsurgical swelling. Because it has blood-thinning abilities, it may also prove useful in preventing heart disease and stroke.

What to Buy: Tablets and capsules are preferred. The dosage of bromelain is based on its milk clotting unit (mcu) activity or on gelatin dissolving units (gdu). One gdu equals 1.5 mcu. Look for supplements that contain at least 2,000 mcu (1,333 gdu) per gram. For example, a 500-mg tablet that contains 2,000 mcu per gram has 1,000 mcu activity.

How to Take: For mild to moderate conditions, take one 500-mg tablet or capsule four times daily. For more severe inflammation or pain, take 3,000 mcu three times daily for several days, then reduce to 2,000 mcu three times daily. Take on an empty stomach when used as an antiinflammatory and with meals when needed as a digestive aid. See individual medical entries for specific dosages.

Possible Side Effects and Precautions: Bromelain is considered to be very safe. Nausea, vomiting, diarrhea, and heavy menstrual bleeding have been reported on very rare occasions. Do not take bromelain if you have gastric ulcers.

Interactions: If you take bromelain and hydrochloric acid, the acid will destroy the enzymes.

CALCIUM Calcium is perhaps best known for its critical role in the formation of bones and teeth, but it also is essential for muscle growth, transmission of nerve impulses, blood clotting, and a regular heartbeat. It helps prevent colon cancer and bone loss (**osteoporosis**) and assists in the structuring of RNA and DNA.

A deficiency of calcium in the diet can cause muscle cramps, heart palpitations (see **heart conditions**), **high blood pressure,** nervousness, tooth decay, rickets, numbness in the legs and/or arms, brittle nails, and aching joints (see **osteoarthritis).** Calcium is sometimes recommended for treatment of **allergies, backache, heart problems, hemorrhoids, menopause, Parkinson's disease,** and **PMS.** Healthy dietary sources of calcium include green leafy vegetables, salmon (with bones), almonds, blackstrap molasses, brewer's yeast, broccoli, kale, kelp, sesame seeds, tofu, and yogurt.

What to Buy: The forms that are best absorbed by the body are calcium citrate-malate (preferred) and calcium carbonate. Both are available in tablets and capsules. Calcium supplements may contain one or more other forms of calcium, such as calcium acetate, gluconate, and lactate. The difference among these forms is the percentage of elemental calcium in the supplement and the absorbency. The higher the percentage of elemental calcium in the supplement, the fewer capsules or tablets you will need to take to reach the optimal calcium intake.

Because calcium and magnesium work closely together in the body, many experts recommend taking the two nutrients together. Combination supplements are available;

some with a ratio of 2:1 (calcium to magnesium) and others at 1:1. Experts disagree as to the best ratio, although 2:1 seems to be preferred.

How to Take: Because calcium is more effective when the body receives it in smaller amounts, divide your daily intake into two or three doses. Take calcium one hour before or two hours after meals and before bedtime, rather than in one dose. See individual medical entries for specific dosages.

Possible Side Effects and Precautions: Taking too much calcium can cause constipation or calcium deposits in the soft tissues. Do not take calcium supplements if you have kidney stones or kidney disease. Avoid Tums with calcium as a calcium source, because the antacid neutralizes the acid needed for calcium absorption. Women with lower estrogen levels (menopausal, postmenopausal, and female athletes) need additional calcium.

You can test the absorption effectiveness of your calcium supplement if you place a calcium pill in a glass of warm water and shake it. Let the mixture sit for twenty-four hours. If the calcium has not dissolved after twenty-four hours, the absorbency rate is poor. Switch to another brand.

Interactions: If you take iron, take your calcium supplement at least two hours after the iron, because calcium inhibits the effectiveness of both nutrients. Excessive calcium interferes with the absorption of zinc, and too much zinc blocks absorption of calcium. Similarly, too much phosphorus and magnesium hinders absorption of calcium. For calcium to be absorbed properly, adequate vitamin D is needed. If you get twenty to thirty minutes of direct sunlight exposure per day, you do not need a vitamin D supplement. The elderly and bedbound patients often need to take a combined calcium and vitamin D supplement.

CARNITINE (L-CARNITINE) Carnitine is a vitaminlike substance that is produced in the body from two other amino acids, lysine and methionine, with the help of several other nutrients. Because its structure is similar to that of an amino acid, it is often classified as such.

L-carnitine stimulates the breakdown of fat to produce energy and prevents the buildup of fat in the heart, skeletal muscles, and liver. Because of its fat-fighting ability carnitine may be supportive in people who have **heart conditions** (e.g., congestive heart failure), **obesity,** or **high blood pressure.** It is also used to help **infertility** in men and to improve muscle strength in people who have neuromuscular conditions. It's been shown that people with some types of muscular dystrophy need greater amounts of carnitine.

Carnitine deficiency is associated with **diabetes,** cirrhosis (see **liver problems**), or **heart conditions** in which oxygen deprivation occurs. Insufficient oxygen supply prevents the heart from storing adequate amounts of carnitine, which leads to an increased risk for angina and heart disease. Some individuals believe it helps **Alzheimer's disease.** A number of people with carnitine deficiency have an inherited condition that hinders carnitine synthesis.

Meat and dairy products contain the highest amounts of carnitine; yet people who eat little or none of these foods will not experience carnitine deficiency if they get sufficient amounts of lysine, which is found in lysine-fortified grains and in vegetables and legumes, and also consume adequate levels of vitamins B_1 and B_6, and iron. Symptoms of carnitine deficiency may include obesity, heart pain, confusion, and muscle weakness.

What to Buy: Free-form L-carnitine, in capsules or tablets, is the preferred form because it is the easiest for the body to absorb. Capsules and tablets come in 250- and 500-mg strength, and some include vitamin C. A powdered form of L-carnitine is also available. Do not get carnitine in any of its other forms: D-carnitine, DL-carnitine, or acetyl–L-carnitine. (The *L* and *D* denote a characteristic of the chemical structure.)

How to Use: As a single supplement: Take 1,000 mg carnitine per day thirty minutes before or after meals. To improve absorption, take carnitine with vitamins B_6 and C. Because a balance among all the amino acids is necessary for the body to function properly, experts usually recommend taking an amino acid complex, which contains all the amino acids, at a different time during the day than when you take carnitine. See individual medical entries for specific dosages.

Possible Side Effects and Precautions: None when taken as directed. At doses 6,000 mg per day or higher, neurological damage may occur. Carnitine should be taken on an empty stomach, as amino acids compete with each other for absorption. Individual amino acids should not be taken for an extended time. Alternate every two months: take for two months, then discontinue for two months, and so on.

Interactions: Carnitine boosts the effectiveness of vitamins C and E.

CAYENNE (CAPSAICIN) Cayenne pepper (*Capsicum frutescens*) is the source of a resinous substance called capsaicin. When taken internally, capsaicin stimulates blood circulation, promotes sweating, and aids digestion. Topical applications are used to reduce inflammation and pain, especially for conditions such as **rheumatoid arthritis, osteoarthritis, psoriasis, shingles,** and **fibromyalgia.** Capsaicin provides temporary relief of pain by depleting small pain fibers of neurotransmitters called substance P. This substance is believed to be the main chemical mediator of pain messages. When the neurotransmitters are depleted, pain cannot be transmitted to the brain.

What to Buy: Look for ointment and lotion containing 0.025 to 0.075 percent capsaicin for external use; tincture for internal use.

How to Use: The ointment and lotion can be applied to unbroken skin. Gloves should be worn or the hands should be washed thoroughly after using capsaicin, because it can cause a burning sensation if it gets into the eyes, mouth, or nose. Tincture—0.3 to 1 mL three times daily. See individual medical entries for specific dosages.

Possible Side Effects and Precautions: Mild burning sensation may be felt at the application site or, in some cases, an allergic reaction may occur. Before the first treatment, apply a minute amount of capsaicin to a small area of skin to test for a possible negative reaction.

CHAMOMILE Chamomile (or camomile) can refer to either the German or Hungarian form (*Matricaria chamomilla*) or to the English or Roman variety (*Anthemis nobilis*). Both species have similar medicinal properties. German chamomile is the most commonly used. The flowers, which contain bioflavonoids and volatile oils, provide the anti-inflammatory and muscle-relaxing properties for which chamomile is known. Chamomile is effective in the treatment of anxiety, **gingivitis,** nervous stomach, and **irritable bowel syndrome.**

What to Buy: The recommended, and most common, forms used are the dried flowers, from which an infusion can be made; prepared tea bags; and tincture. Chamomile is also available as tablets and capsules.

How to Use: To prepare an infusion, add 1 Tbs dried flowers (or 1 prepared tea bag) to 1 cup boiling water. Allow to steep for ten to fifteen minutes. Drink 3 to 4 cups daily. Other standard dosages include 4 to 6 mL tincture three times daily between meals or 2 to 3 g capsules or tablets three times daily between meals. See individual medical entries for specific dosages.

Possible Side Effects and Precautions: Side effects are rare. If you have allergies to ragweed aster, or chrysanthemum, however, do not use chamomile. Chamomile is safe to use during pregnancy and lactation.

CHASTE BERRY The chaste tree (*Vitex agnus-castus*), also known as vitex, is a small shrub that grows in Europe and in the southern United States. The berries of this shrub have the ability to restore the balance of estrogen and progesterone in women, which makes it an effective treatment for symptoms of **endometriosis, fibrocystic breast disease, infertility, PMS,** and **menopause.**

What to Buy: The preferred forms are tincture, capsules (containing dried herb), and the berries. It is also available as a powder.

How to Use: To prepare an infusion using the berries, add 1 tsp ripe berries to 1 cup boiling water and let steep, covered, for ten to fifteen minutes. Drink 3 cups per day. Other general dosages include 500 to 1,000 mg daily or dried herb capsules, and 1 to 2 dropperfuls tincture daily. Benefits are usually noticeable by day ten, but for best results, take chaste tree for six months or longer. See individual medical entries for specific dosages.

Possible Side Effects and Precautions: Do not use this herb while using birth control pills. Stop taking chaste tree by the third month of pregnancy, as it stimulates breast milk production.

CHONDROITIN SULFATE. (See glucosamine sulfate.)

CHROMIUM Chromium is an essential trace mineral that helps the body maintain healthy levels of cholesterol and blood sugar. Many people take chromium as an aid to lose fat and gain lean muscle, but research has not confirmed the validity of these uses. Chromium is found in brewer's yeast, beer, brown rice, grains, and cereals, although much of this mineral can be lost during processing. Supplements of chromium are taken to treat **diabetes, acne, psoriasis, and glaucoma** and to help with weight loss and **obesity.**

What to Buy: The preferred forms are chelated tablets, such as chelated chromium picolinate, which is chromium chelated with the natural amino acid metabolite called picolinate. Picolinate allows chromium to enter the cells more efficiently. Another form, chromium polynicotinate (chromium chelated to niacin), is also effective. Chromium is often part of a high-quality multivitamin-mineral formula.

How to Use: The U.S. National Academy of Science recommends 50 to 200 mcg per day. Some experts prescribe up to 300 mcg daily. Take with food and with vitamin C. See individual medical conditions for specific dosages.

Possible Side Effects and Precautions: No toxicity has been noted at doses of 50 to 300 mcg per day. Some people develop a rash or feel light-headed when taking chromium. If taken regularly at levels of 1,000 mcg or higher, kidney and liver damage is likely. Because chromium can affect blood sugar levels, people with diabetes should consult their physician before taking chromium supplements.

Interactions: Vitamin C helps increase the absorption of chromium.

COENZYME Q10 The other name for this vitaminlike substance is ubiquinone, a term that indicates (from the word *ubiquitous*) the fact that it is found in nearly every cell in the body. Coenzyme Q10 is most concentrated in the mitochondria of cells, where energy is produced, and is most abundant in the heart. Energy production is this enzyme's main role: it helps transform food into ATP, or adenosine triphosphate, the energy that makes the body function. In fact, coenzyme Q10 has a role in 95 percent of the energy generated by the body. It is also a potent antioxidant that has the ability to interfere with histamine, a substance that causes symptoms of asthma and other respiratory conditions.

Much is still unknown about coenzyme Q10. Deficiency appears to be caused by problems with synthesizing the nutrient rather than low intake from diet. Low levels of coenzyme Q10 are often seen in people who have **heart problems** (including angina, congestive heart failure, and mitral valve prolapse), **AIDS,** and **gingivitis** (inflammation of the gums), and in the elderly. Coenzyme Q10 is used to treat people in all these populations as well as those with yeast infections (see **vaginitis**), **allergies, cancer, chronic fatigue syndrome, diabetes, high blood pressure, liver problems, Raynaud's syndrome, obesity, Alzheimer's disease,** and muscular dystrophy.

Coenzyme Q10 is found in mackerel, sardines, spinach, peanuts, and salmon. It is widely used in Japan to treat heart disease and high blood pressure and to boost the immune system.

What to Buy: Softgel capsules are the preferred form because they are assimilated better than the other available forms—dry capsules and tablets. Get softgels that contain vitamin E, as this combination helps preserve the coenzyme Q10. The softgels should be bright yellow to orange; these colors indicate that the formulation is pure. Coenzyme Q10 is fairly expensive. Be aware that there are some inferior "bargain" brands on the market, which lure you with reduced prices but which also contain fillers—wheat, corn meal, yeast, eggs, sugars, and/or milk derivatives—in place of the enzyme.

How to Use: There is no DRI for coenzyme Q10. Recommended dosage levels range from 30 to 150 mg per day, although individuals with specific health problems usually take higher doses. Consult your health-care provider to determine the best dosage for you. To optimize the benefits and absorption of coenzyme Q10, take the supplements with a little fat, such as peanut butter or oil, or take a coenzyme Q10 supplement that contains vitamin E. See individual medical entries for specific dosages.

Possible Side Effects and Precautions: Individuals with congestive heart failure who take coenzyme Q10 should not stop taking the supplement without consulting their physician. Do not take this supplement if you are pregnant or breast-feeding. Because coenzyme Q10 is perishable, keep it away from light and heat; it deteriorates in temperatures greater than 115 degrees F.

COPPER This mineral has an important role in the formation of bone, red blood cells, and hemoglobin, as it is necessary for the proper absorption of iron. It also plays a part in energy production, regulation of heart rate and blood pressure, fertility, taste sensitivity, skin and hair coloring, and the healing process. Supplementation with copper may be helpful for some people with **rheumatoid arthritis** or **cataracts.**

Copper deficiency is uncommon, but it can occur in people who take a zinc supplement and do not increase their intake of copper, because zinc, as well as vitamin C and calcium, can interfere with copper absorption. It may also occur in people who have Crohn's disease, celiac disease, albinism, or infants who were not breast-fed. Signs of deficiency include brittle hair, anemia, high blood pressure, heart arrhythmias, infertility, and skeletal defects.

Although most people consume less than the DRI of copper, supplementation is recommended only for people who are taking zinc supplements, either alone or as part of a multivitamin-mineral formula. If your multiple contains copper, then you probably have adequate protection against deficiency. Copper is found in seafood, blackstrap molasses, nuts, seeds, green vegetables, black pepper, cocoa, and water that is carried via copper pipes.

What to Buy: Look for a multivitamin-mineral that has copper. If you need a copper supplement, look for copper aspartate, copper citrate, or copper picolinate.

How to Use: Most people get sufficient copper in their multivitamin-mineral supplement. If you need additional copper, take 1.5 to 3 mg daily with food. See individual medical entries for specific dosages.

Possible Side Effects: When taken at recommended dosages, no side effects are expected. At high doses (10 mg or more), nausea, vomiting, muscle pain, and stomach pain may occur. Some experts believe excessive copper may be linked with autism and hyperactivity. Excessive copper may also cause damage to joint tissues.

Precautions: People with Wilson's disease should not take copper supplements. If your drinking water travels through copper pipes, check the copper content of your water before taking a supplement. Women who are pregnant or who are taking birth control pills should ask their physician before taking copper supplements.

Interactions: Copper improves absorption and use of iron.

DANDELION The dandelion (*Taraxacum officinale*), often regarded as a weed, has extremely high levels of vitamin A and good levels of vitamins C, D, and various B vitamins, plus iron, silicon, magnesium, manganese, and potassium. Its high iron content makes it a good treatment for **anemia,** and its ability to promote the flow of bile in the liver makes it a possible therapy choice for hepatitis and jaundice (see **liver problems**). Women with **PMS** often take dandelion to help relieve water retention. The rich level of potassium in the leaves makes dandelion the only known potassium-sparing diuretic. (Diuretics typically deplete the body of potassium, which is a problem with most diuretic drugs.) Dandelion is also used to treat **canker sores, eczema,** and **constipation.** The bitter components known as sesquiteropene lactones, found in both the roots and leaves, are responsible for dandelion's healing qualities.

What to Buy: Recommended forms include fluid extract, powdered solid extract, dried root, and dried leaves. Also available as tablets, capsules, and tincture. The alcohol-based tincture should be avoided because an extremely high dosage is required to be effective.

How to Take: To prepare the dried root as a decoction, simmer 1 Tbs in 8 oz boiling water for ten minutes; strain and drink up to 3 cups per day. Other general dosages include 4 to 8 mL (1 to 2 tsp) fluid extract and 500 to 1,000 mg powdered extract. See individual medical entries for specific dosages.

Possible Side Effects and Precautions: When used to treat gallstones, gastritis, or stomach ulcer, dandelion should be used under supervision of a health-care professional. If you gather fresh dandelion leaves to dry for infusions, note that some people are allergic to the latex in the fresh leaves and experience a rash.

DHEA Dehydroepiandrosterone (DHEA) is a hormone produced by the adrenal glands, which is eventually converted into other hormones in the body, such as progesterone, testosterone, and estrogen. Because DHEA is a naturally occurring substance, it cannot be patented, which discourages drug companies from spending money on research. Synthetic versions are available, however, and currently under scrutiny for treatment of AIDS and lupus.

Because DHEA levels are highest in persons who are younger than forty and decline rapidly thereafter, many people believe it is an antiaging agent. This claim has not been proved or disproved, yet the supplement has gained much popularity for this purpose, as well as for people with **Alzheimer's disease.** DHEA is credited with enhancing sex drive, helping **erectile problems (impotence),** treating **obesity,** relieving **rheumatoid arthritis,** reducing stress, boosting the immune system, improving memory, and helping in the treatment of cancer, Parkinson's disease, and diabetes, although its effectiveness in these conditions has not been proven.

What to Buy: Sublingual capsules and liquid are the preferred forms; tablets and capsules are also available. DHEA can be purchased in both nonprescription and prescription strength. Some products are sold as "natural" DHEA precursors derived from wild yam. Despite claims by some manufacturers, wild yam products do not contain DHEA, nor do they transform into DHEA in the body. To make this conversion wild yam must undergo a chemical conversion process in the laboratory. Most products, however, are processed from diosgenin, a substance extracted from wild yam.

How to Use: Because DHEA is a hormone, its use as a supplement is controversial. Even among its proponents there is disagreement about the best dosage. Some suggest 2 to 10 mg per day; others say up to 50 mg is safe. Most agree that women should take dosages one third to one half lower than men. The possibility of liver damage prompts some physicians to recommend taking a basic antioxidant regimen (vitamins C and E and selenium) along with DHEA to help prevent liver problems. It is best to consult with a professional knowledgeable about nutrition before taking DHEA and, after starting it, to have your blood taken periodically to monitor DHEA blood levels.

Possible Side Effects: Minor side effects include acne, mood swings, fatigue, insomnia, enlarged breasts in men, and unwanted body hair in women, such as facial hair. Some experts believe liver damage is possible. Because no long-term (more than six months) studies have been done with DHEA, the benefits or disadvantages of prolonged use are unknown.

Precautions: Take DHEA only under medical supervision. Individuals with a personal or family history of any hormone-related cancer, such as prostate or breast cancer, should not take DHEA, because DHEA is a precursor of estrogen and testosterone. Some experts believe that taking high levels of DHEA interferes with the body's ability to naturally synthesize the hormone.

Interactions: If you are taking estrogen, DHEA may affect your dosage requirements. DHEA also may interact with over-the-counter or prescription drugs, nutritional supplements, or herbal remedies.

DONG QUAI This Chinese herbal supplement, also known as angelica root (*Angelica sinensis*), has a long history of use for gynecological problems. It has proved effective in the treatment of amenorrhea (lack of menstruation) and menstrual cramps, **PMS,** poor blood circulation, **endometriosis, fibrocystic breast disease, menopause,** blurred vision, and heart palpitations. Some acupuncturists inject the herb into acupuncture points as a treatment for pain of **osteoarthritis, rheumatoid arthritis,** and neuralgia.

Dong quai is believed to be effective because it balances women's hormone levels. It is also beneficial for people with high blood pressure and poor circulation. Dong quai is often mixed with other Chinese herbs to treat specific conditions.

What to Buy: Fluid extract, tincture, and powdered root in capsules are the preferred forms; also available in tablets.

How to Use: Typical dosage for the fluid extract is 1 mL three times daily; for the tincture, 4 mL three times daily;

and the powdered root, 1 to 2 g three times daily. The powdered root can be taken in capsules or used to make an infusion. Steep 1 to 2 g in 8 oz boiled water for ten minutes. Drink 3 cups daily. Dosages of powdered root can range from 500 mg to 4 g or more per day, depending on the condition being treated. See individual medical entries for specific dosages.

Possible Side Effects and Precautions: Dong quai is safe when taken as directed. In large doses, however, it can cause diarrhea or abdominal bloating. Do not take during pregnancy.

ECHINACEA Echinacea (*Echinacea purpurea*) is a wildflower also known as purple coneflower. It was widely used by Native Americans and was quickly adopted by the settlers for many uses, including common cold, syphilis, and snakebites. Today it is a popular and effective treatment for **common cold and flu, bronchitis, sinusitus,** yeast infections (see **vaginitis**), **canker sores,** Crohn's disease (see **inflammatory bowel disease**), and **ear infections.**

Echinacea contains several beneficial ingredients. Echinacoside is believed to have antibiotic properties, while echinacein appears to limit the actions of invading bacteria and viruses.

What to Buy: Recommended—according to Michael Murray, ND, the best echinacea product to buy is the fresh-pressed juice (not the same as a fluid extract) of *E. purpurea* standardized for a minimum of 2.4 percent beta-1,2-fructofuranosides. This form, however, is not always readily available. Other recommended forms include solid (dry powdered) extract standardized for 3.5 percent echinacoside, fluid extract, tincture, and freeze-dried plant. Also available is dried root, which can be used to make decoctions.

How to Use: General dosages include any of the following three times daily: 3 to 4 mL (^{3}/$_4$ to 1 tsp) tincture; 1 to 2 mL (^{1}/$_4$ to ^{1}/$_2$ tsp) fluid extract; 300 mg solid dry powdered extract (3.5 percent echinacoside); 325 to 650 mg freeze-dried plant; or 2 to 3 mL (^{1}/$_2$ to ^{3}/$_4$ tsp) juice of *E. purpurea*. To make a decoction, boil 2 tsp dried root in 8 oz water and simmer covered for fifteen minutes. Drink up to 3 cups daily.

Possible Side Effects and Precautions: Generally, do not use echinacea for longer than two weeks. If you are treating a chronic immune-system condition, the usual recommendation is eight weeks of treatment followed by one week off. Consult with your physician before taking echinacea if you are pregnant or nursing. Combine echinacea with an equal amount of uva ursi to treat cystitis (see **urinary-tract infections**).

EPHEDRA Ephedra (*Ephedra sinica*) is an herb that is used to relieve respiratory conditions such as **allergies, bronchitis,** and asthma, to control weight, and to increase energy. Of the three active ingredients in ephedra, the one that can cause adverse reactions is ephedrine (see below). Because of these side effects many professionals discourage the use of ephedra or products containing it for weight loss (see **obesity**). Consult your health-care provider before using ephedra.

What to Buy: Look for the fluid extract standardized for 10 percent alkaloid content; also standardized tablets and dried bulk herb if available.

How to Use: The general dosage for an extract standardized at 10 percent alkaloids is 125 to 250 mg three times daily. For nonstandardized tablets and bulk herb used to make infusions, the average alkaloid content is 1 to 3 percent, which means you need to take higher doses. To prepare an infusion using standardized dry herb, use 1 to 2 tsp dried ephedra in 8 oz water, simmer for ten to fifteen minutes. Drink up to 2 cups per day.

Possible Side Effects: Nonserious side effects include dry mouth, insomnia, nervousness, headache, and dizziness; more serious ones include increased blood pressure and heart rate, and heart palpitations. Stop ephedra immediately and call your physician if you experience any serious reactions.

Precautions: Do not take ephedra if you have heart disease, diabetes, high blood pressure, anxiety, hyperthyroidism, or glaucoma, or if you are pregnant. If you are taking any medications, do not use ephedra until you talk with your doctor.

EVENING PRIMROSE OIL Evening primrose oil is the best food source for an essential fatty acid called gamma-linolenic acid (GLA). GLA converts to prostaglandin E1 (PGE1), a hormonelike substance that helps dilate blood vessels, thin the blood, and reduce inflammation. These properties help make evening primrose oil useful in the prevention of **endometriosis, fibrocystic breast disease, heart problems, irritable bowel syndrome, menopause, multiple sclerosis, PMS, osteoarthritis,** and brittle hair and nails. It is also an effective treatment for **acne, dandruff, depression, migraine, psoriasis, seborrheic dermatitis,** and pain. For women with PMS evening primrose oil is especially helpful in relieving hot flashes, cramping, and bloating, because the prostaglandins help maintain the hormone balance.

Most people in the United States are deficient in GLA. Those most likely to have low levels of GLA include people with diabetes, **eczema,** or **PMS,** all of whom may have an inability to properly produce GLA.

What to Buy: Recommended—softgel capsules and liquid (oil).

How to Use: Although no optimal intake level has been determined, experts generally recommend taking 3,000 to 6,000 mg of evening primrose oil daily, which supplies 270 to 360 mg of GLA. You need to take evening primrose oil for about thirty days before you will notice its benefits.

Possible Side Effects and Precautions: Side effects are not common; headache, nausea, and rash are possible. These reactions usually disappear if you reduce the dosage. Evening primrose oil may increase mania in people with manic depression and exacerbate temporal lobe epilepsy. Women who have estrogen-related breast cancer should avoid this supplement because it promotes the production of estrogen.

Interactions: To make prostaglandin E1, the body also requires magnesium, zinc, vitamin C, niacin, and vitamin B_6. Some experts recommend taking these supplements along with evening primrose oil.

FENUGREEK Fenugreek (*Trigonella foenum-graecum*) is a member of the legume family and is one of the world's oldest medicinal herbs. In many parts of the world it is used as a food and a spice, as well as for medicinal purposes. Conditions that often respond to fenugreek include digestive problems, **constipation, diabetes,** high cholesterol (see **atherosclerosis**), cough and sore throat, and skin injuries. Consult your physician before using fenugreek for diabetes.

The seeds of the fenugreek plant contain several substances that are responsible for its healing powers. One is mucilage, a gelatinous substance that is soothing to the digestive system and respiratory tract. Another is a group of alkaloids, which help in the treatment of diabetes by reducing the amount of sugar in the urine and improving glucose tolerance. Other components found in fenugreek include all of the B vitamins, vitamin A, and vitamin D.

What to Buy: Recommended forms are defatted seed powder or debitterized seeds, especially for diabetes. The powder is available in capsules. The tincture is also a preferred form, although it is not always readily available.

How to Use: Fenugreek seeds are bitter, therefore debitterized seeds are easier to take. They can be added to food or made into an infusion. To prepare an infusion, boil 8 oz water and add 2 tsp ground fenugreek seeds. Simmer for ten minutes. Drink up to 3 cups per day. Add honey, sugar, or lemon extract to improve the flavor. Other general dosages include 15 to 90 g (capsules) once daily with food. Take the tincture according to package directions. See individual medical entries for specific dosages.

Possible Side Effects and Precautions: Fenugreek is very safe when taken at recommended doses. If more than 100 g per day is used, nausea and intestinal upset may occur. If uterine contractions occur, call your doctor immediately. If pregnant, do not take fenugreek because of possible uterine contractions.

Interactions: If you combine fenugreek with other herbs, you may need to decrease the dosage.

FEVERFEW Feverfew (*Tanacetum parthenium* or *Chrysanthemum parthenium*) is a flowering plant that has been used since ancient times to treat **migraine,** inflammation, and pain associated with menstruation. In the 1970s British researchers discovered that feverfew leaves are effective in the treatment of migraine. They attribute its pain-relieving ability to parthenolide. This chemical prevents substances that cause inflammation from entering the bloodstream and traveling to the blood vessels in the brain, where they appear to be at least partially responsible for migraine pain.

What to Buy: The most effective forms are the fresh leaves or any standardized extract, tincture, or capsule at 0.40 to 0.66 percent parthenolide. Some combination forms contain Siberian ginseng, ginkgo, or meadowsweet. Also available are tablets.

How to Use: Chewing fresh leaves (two to three medium-sized leaves per day) provides the best relief, but they are very bitter. The leaves can be put into a sandwich to make them more palatable. To make an infusion with the dried bulk herb, add 2 to 3 tsp dried herb to 8 oz boiling water and allow to steep for five to ten minutes. Drink 2 to 3 cups daily. See the entry for **headache and migraine** for additional dosage information.

Possible Side Effects and Precautions: Chewing feverfew may cause sores in the mouth or stomach upset. Pregnant women should not take feverfew, because it may cause uterine contractions. Do not take feverfew if you have a blood-clotting disorder or are taking anticoagulant medication. Allow two to three months of taking feverfew daily before results become apparent.

FOLIC ACID Folic acid, also known as vitamin B$_9$, folate, and folacin, plays many crucial roles in maintaining health. It is a vital ingredient in the makeup of RNA and DNA— the body's genetic material. Women who are planning to become or who are pregnant need adequate levels of folic acid (see p. 42) because it is instrumental in preventing most neural-tube birth defects as well as congenital abnormalities (also see **infertility**). It helps prevent heart disease by keeping homocysteine (an amino acid) levels down, and it has a key role in keeping the skin, nails, nerves, mucous membranes, hair, and blood healthy. Supplements may be beneficial for people with **anemia, atherosclerosis,** Crohn's disease (see **inflammatory bowel disease**), **depression, diarrhea, gingivitis, gout, osteoporosis,** or skin problems such as vitiligo.

Folic acid is found in avocados, beans, beets, celery, citrus, fortified cereal, green leafy vegetables, nuts, orange juice, seeds, and peas. A deficiency is most likely to occur among people who have gastrointestinal or malabsorption disorders, women who take oral contraceptives, pregnant women who are not taking vitamin supplements, alcoholics, and teenagers who have a poor diet. Signs of deficiency include headache, loss of appetite, diarrhea, fatigue, paleness, insomnia, and an inflamed, red tongue.

What to Buy: Look for multivitamin-mineral supplements with folic acid, preferably in the form of folinic acid (5-methyl-tetra-hydrofolate), because this is the most bioactive form; or take the individual supplement, available in tablets.

How to Use: Average daily therapeutic intake of 400 mcg is recommended for adults; 400 to 800 mcg for people with cancer and for women who are or who could become pregnant. The body needs folic acid to properly use vitamin B_{12}. If you are deficient in vitamin B_{12}, intake of 1,000 mcg folic acid may be needed to treat the anemia caused by the B_{12} deficiency. Consult a health professional who is knowledgeable in vitamin B_{12} deficient anemia.

Possible Side Effects and Precautions: Folic acid is considered safe and there are no known side effects. High doses of folic acid may hide the symptoms of vitamin B_{12} deficiency. If you have any reason to suspect a B_{12} deficiency, consult with a knowledgeable health professional before starting a folic acid supplement program.

Interactions: Antacids and proteolytic enzymes can interfere with folic acid absorption; thus it is advisable to take a folic acid supplement if you are taking these substances.

GARLIC One of the oldest and most commonly used medicinal plants is garlic (*Allium sativum*). It contains sulfur compounds, including allicin, ajoene, allyl sulfides, and vinyldithins, which are responsible for garlic's antibiotic actions. Conditions that respond to garlic intake include **ath-**

erosclerosis, AIDS, bronchitis, heart problems, diarrhea, diverticulitis, herpes, high blood pressure, colds and flu, ear infections, irritable bowel syndrome, prostate problems, and yeast infections (see vaginitis). Regular intake of garlic reduces the risk of cancer of the colon, stomach, and esophagus and helps inhibit the growth of some cancers, including skin and breast.

What to Buy: Look for products standardized to provide up to 5,000 mcg allicin daily. To avoid smelling like garlic, odor-free, enteric-coated tablets and capsules are available; garlic oil and tinctures are also on the market.

How to Use: General dosage for tablets and capsules is 400 to 500 mg one to two times per day (up to 5,000 mcg allicin). For tinctures, take 2 to 4 mL (5 to 25 drops) three times per day. See individual medical entries for specific dosages.

Possible Side Effects and Precautions: People who are sensitive to garlic may experience flatulence or heartburn. Garlic has anticlotting properties; therefore, if you are taking anticoagulant drugs, do not take garlic supplements without first consulting your physician.

GERMANIUM Germanium is a trace element (an essential substance found in minute levels in the body) found naturally in garlic, sea algae, aloe vera, shiitake mushrooms, Siberian ginseng, and barley. It is classified as an immunostimulant because it activates the immune system and promotes the production of gamma-interferon, an anticancer, antiviral substance. This naturally occurring element does not appear to have a significant impact on health, but synthetic organic compounds developed by Japanese researchers do. One of the most common of these compounds is called Ge-132, or organic germanium sesquioxide.

Organic germanium compounds fight viral infections,

help prevent cancer, improve circulation, balance bodily functions, and boost the immune system. These properties make it effective in the treatment of **AIDS, cancer, depression, fibrocystic breast disease, glaucoma, gout, heart problems,** high cholesterol (see **atherosclerosis**), **liver problems, osteoarthritis, Raynaud's disease,** and **rheumatoid arthritis.** It also is a fast-acting painkiller and improves circulation to the brain. Germanium works by attaching itself to oxygen molecules, which deliver the mineral to the body's cells and enhance the oxygen supply. The increased oxygen allows the body to rid itself of poisons and toxins.

What to Buy: The recommended form is colloidal liquid. Also available in powder, granules, capsules, and tablets. Germanium is expensive and not as readily available as many other supplements.

How to Take: Colloidal liquid can be taken under the tongue or mixed in juice or water ($^1/_2$ tsp in 6 oz liquid) in the morning or as indicated. The average dosage for other forms is 75 to 150 mg daily. Take with water on an empty stomach. See individual medical entries for specific dosages.

Possible Side Effects and Precautions: Minor skin eruptions, which disappear within a few days, occur in a small number of people. Loose stools may occur if high doses of germanium (more than 400 mg daily) are taken for more than thirty days.

GINGER The dried rhizome of this perennial plant has been used for thousands of years for various gastrointestinal problems, such as bloating, loose stools, **flatulence, heartburn, nausea,** and vomiting, and for treatment of inflammatory conditions, such as **rheumatoid arthritis.** Ginger (*Zingiber officinale*) is also effective in the treatment of menstrual cramps and **migraine** headache. The volatile oils in dried rhizome of ginger, including gingerols, shogaols, zingiberene, and bisabolene, are responsible for its healing powers.

What to Buy: Recommended forms are dried root powder and fresh root. Also available in tablets, capsules, tincture, and prepared tea bags.

How to Take: The dried root powder can be added to liquids or food. To make a decoction, simmer 1 to 2 tsp dried root powder in 1 cup water for five to ten minutes; take as needed. To make a fresh root decoction, simmer 1 tsp grated fresh root in 1 cup water for fifteen minutes. Strain and take as needed. See individual medical entries for specific dosages.

Possible Side Effects and Precautions: Some people experience temporary heartburn. Long-term use of ginger during pregnancy is not recommended. If you have a history of gallstones, consult your physician before taking ginger.

Interactions: If combining ginger with other herbs, you may need to reduce the amount of ginger.

GINKGO The fan-shaped leaves of the ginkgo tree (*Ginkgo biloba*) have been highly regarded for their medicinal value for thousands of years. Ginkgo is effective against vascular diseases and improves circulation, especially to the lower legs and feet and to the brain, where it may improve memory and concentration. Conditions treated with ginkgo include vertigo, **Alzheimer's disease, depression, glaucoma, erectile dysfunction (impotence), macular degeneration, multiple sclerosis,** leg ulcers, **Raynaud's syndrome,** and obesity. Ginkgo contains various bioflavonoids, including quercetin and flavoglycosides, which appear to be the plant's healing compounds.

What to Buy: Recommended—a standardized extract at 24 percent flavoglycosides and 6 percent terpene lactones. Also available in standardized capsules, tablets, and dry bulk. Do not buy nonstandardized products, as there is extreme variation in the content of its active ingredients.

How to Use: Dosages range from 120 to 160 mg two to three times daily for tablets and capsules, and 40 to 80 mg three times daily for extract. It takes at least two weeks before results are apparent. See individual medical entries for specific dosages.

Possible Side Effects and Precautions: If you experience diarrhea, vomiting, nausea, irritability, or restlessness when taking ginkgo, consult your health-care practitioner to determine if you should reduce the dosage or stop taking the herb. Do not take ginkgo if you have a clotting disorder or if you are nursing or pregnant.

GINSENG Ginseng is an herb that is available in several species: Siberian ginseng (*Eleutherococcus senticosus*), American ginseng (*Panax quinquefolium*), Chinese or Korean ginseng (*Panax ginseng*), and Japanese ginseng (*Panax japonicum*). The most common and widely used is Chinese ginseng.

All forms of ginseng are often used to battle fatigue and increase energy levels; thus ginseng is usually regarded as a general tonic. Ginseng has the ability to regulate blood sugar fluctuations, and to stimulate circulation. When taken in low doses it can increase blood pressure; at higher doses it reduces it. This ability to adapt to the body's needs places ginseng in the category of "adaptogens," substances that regulate and normalize the body's systems.

Both the Siberian and American ginsengs are commonly used to treat inflammation, **chronic fatigue syndrome,** fatigue, and stress. Asian ginseng typically is taken for shortness of breath, fever, vomiting, and **erectile dysfunction** (impotence). The active ingredients in American and Asian ginseng are known as ginsenosides, while those in Siberian ginseng are called eleutherosides.

What to Buy: Look for American and Asian ginseng products that are standardized for 5 to 9 percent ginsenosides, or Siberian ginseng standardized for more than 1 percent eleutherosides. Look for name brands with a reputation for quality. Suggested forms are any reputable standardized powdered or liquid extract, tincture, capsules, or fresh root. Also available are granules and tablets. Many manufacturers produce supplements that contain some ginseng as part of the formula; however, the levels are usually too low to have any therapeutic impact. Siberian ginseng tends to be less expensive than the other varieties.

How to Use: To make a decoction using American or Asian ginseng, take 1 oz fresh root and boil it in 8 oz water for fifteen minutes. Drink up to 2 cups per day. Typical dosages range from 250 to 500 mg one to two times daily for capsules and 10 to 20 mL ($2^{1}/_{2}$ to 5 tsp) three times daily for tincture. If taking American or Asian ginseng for an extended time, follow each fifteen- to twenty-day course of treatment with a two-week no-treatment period.

For Siberian ginseng—typical dosages include any of the following three times a day: 10 to 20 mL tincture; 100 to 200 mg dry powdered extract; 2 to 4 mL fluid extract. For long-term treatment, follow each sixty-day course with a two- to three-week no-treatment period. See individual medical entries for specific dosages.

Possible Side Effects and Precautions: All forms of ginseng may cause the same types of side effects, including headache, insomnia, breast tenderness, anxiety, and rash. More serious reactions may include asthma attacks, increased blood pressure, and heart palpitations.

GLUCOSAMINE (SULFATE) Glucosamine is a substance found naturally in the body. Its primary function is to provide the joints with the material necessary to produce glycosaminoglycan, a critical ingredient in cartilage. It also helps in the formation of tendons, skin, bones, nails, and ligaments. Glucosamine sulfate is the artificially produced version of the natural substance. It is used to treat osteoarthritis and other types of joint pain and stiffness, and reportedly is helpful for **kidney stones** as well.

Studies indicate that glucosamine relieves the pain and stiffness associated with **osteoarthritis** by stimulating the cells that produce glycosaminoglycans and proteoglycans, another substance important in building cartilage. Glucosamine is also credited with antiinflammatory properties and may be a safe, reliable alternative to aspirin and other anti-inflammatory drugs, which often cause dangerous side effects, such as stomach bleeding and stomach ulcers.

Another substance produced by the body that is a significant component of cartilage is chondroitin sulfate. Its function in cartilage is to provide structure, retain nutrients and water, and allow molecules to pass through. Because it is able to perform these functions, some experts say chondroitin may benefit people with **osteoarthritis.**

Use of chondroitin for arthritis is controversial, however. Although the absorption rate of **glucosamine** sulfate is 90 percent or better, that of chondroitin is 13 percent at best. That's because chondroitin molecules are much bigger than those of glucosamine and so have little success being absorbed or even reaching cartilage cells. This situation has led some researchers to suggest that chondroitin is most effective when it is combined with glucosamine. Although many patients and doctors believe chondroitin works synergistically with glucosamine sulfate to relieve arthritis pain and inflammation, this has not been proven scientifically.

Experts have not identified a specific healthy level of chondroitin in the body. However, many do believe reduced amounts may be characteristic of people with osteoarthritis or other forms of arthritis. Studies have shown that chondroitin may promote healing of bone and may restore joint function, which makes it a possible treatment for osteoarthritis.

What to Buy: Capsules; some glucosamine products also contain chondroitin sulfate. When buying a combination product, look for brands in which the glucosamine-to-chondroitin dose ratio is 5:4 (e.g., 500 mg glucosamine and 400 mg chondroitin).

How to Use: For treatment of arthritis the typical dosage for glucosamine alone is one 500-mg capsule three times daily. For combination products dosage is dependent upon body weight. If you weigh less than 120 pounds, take 1,000 mg glucosamine and 800 mg chondroitin; 120 to 200 pounds, 1,500 mg glucosamine and 1,200 mg chondroitin; and more than 200 pounds, 2,000 mg glucosamine and 1,600 mg chondroitin.

Possible Side Effects and Precautions: Occasionally individuals experience minor side effects with glucosamine, including heartburn, diarrhea, nausea, indigestion, and stomach upset. Some glucosamine formulations contain sodium chloride (salt), which should be avoided by people with high blood pressure. If taking chondroitin, dosages greater than 10 g per day may cause nausea.

GOLDENSEAL Goldenseal (*Hydrastis canadensis*) is an herb whose root and rhizome are valued for their antiinflammatory and antimicrobial properties. It also has the ability to aid digestion and dry up secretions.

The Native Americans used goldenseal to treat various types of inflammation and irritations of the urinary, respiratory, and digestive tracts. Today it is still used for these conditions, including **athlete's foot,** infectious **diarrhea, flatulence, gingivitis, herpes, sinusitis, urinary-tract infections,** and **ulcers.** Berberine, the main alkaloid found in goldenseal, is responsible for the plant's antimicrobial action, especially against *Escherichia coli, Salmonella typhi,* and the species *Chlamydia.* Other alkaloids, including hydrastine, berberastine, and canadine, also have some medicinal value.

What to Buy: Recommended are any forms standardized for 8 to 12 percent alkaloid content, including powdered dry extract, fluid extract, tincture, and capsules. Also available as dried root to make decoctions.

How to Use: General dosages include 4 to 6 g in capsules daily in divided doses, and 4 to 6 mL tincture daily in divided doses. To make a decoction, pour 8 oz boiling water over 2 tsp goldenseal powder and steep covered for ten to fifteen minutes. Drink up to 3 cups daily. Do not use goldenseal for more than three weeks continuously. After three weeks, stop treatment for at least two weeks before starting again.

Possible Side Effects and Precautions: In high doses goldenseal may cause nausea, diarrhea, or irritation of the skin, throat, vagina, or mouth. Stop taking the herb if any of these reactions occur. Do not take goldenseal if you are pregnant or nursing, or if you have diabetes, glaucoma, high blood pressure, heart disease, or if you've had a stroke.

GREEN TEA Green tea is derived from the same plant as are black and oolong teas, *Camellia sinensis.* The difference lies in how the tea leaves are prepared. Green tea maintains all of its active constituents because the leaves are not fermented, as are those of both black and oolong teas. These active components, called polyphenols, appear to be responsible for green tea's beneficial properties. These include the ability to protect against **heart disease** by lowering blood pressure, lowering total cholesterol levels, and reducing platelet aggregation (the clumping of blood cells that may lead to clotting). Green tea has also demonstrated the ability to reduce the risk of some **cancers,** especially esophageal cancer, and to fight bacteria, including the type that causes **gingivitis** and bad breath.

What to Buy: Look for prepared tea or capsules with an extract standardized for 80 percent total polyphenol and 55 percent epigallocatechin gallate (a type of polyphenol). If you want to avoid the caffeine, purchase decaffeinated varieties.

How to Use: To make tea, pour 8 oz boiling water over 1 tsp green tea leaves and steep for three minutes. Drink up to 5 cups daily, preferably with meals. Of capsules, take 500 mg daily.

Possible Side Effects and Precautions: Drinking large amounts of tea may cause insomnia, anxiety, or restlessness because of the caffeine content. According to Michael Murray, ND, green tea typically does not cause these symptoms. You may want to use a decaffeinated brand if you are sensitive to caffeine.

HAWTHORN Hawthorn (*Crataegus laeviata,* also *Crataegus oxyacantha, Crataegus monogyna*) is a European shrub whose leaves, flowers, and fruit are often used to treat **heart problems,** including angina, cardiac arrhythmias, heart palpitations, congestive heart failure, and **atherosclerosis.** The compounds present in hawthorn that give this herb its healing properties include quercetin, oligomeric procyanidine, and vitexin. These ingredients help treat **high blood pressure,** improve contractions of the heart, enhance coronary-artery blood flow, lower blood pressure, and reduce production of angiotensin II, a substance that constricts blood vessels.

What to Buy: The preferred form is the extract standardized for total bioflavonoid content of 2.2 percent or oligomeric procyanidins of 18.75 percent. Look for tincture, fluid extract, capsules, and dried leaves and berries.

How to Use: Typical dosage ranges are 4 to 5 mL tincture; 80 to 300 mg capsules; or 1 to 2 mL fluid extract, three times daily. To make an infusion of the dried leaves or berries, add 3 to 5 g of herb to 8 oz boiling water and allow to steep ten minutes. Drink up to three cups daily. Always consult with your physician before starting hawthorn. Allow one to two months for the effects to be noticeable.

Possible Side Effects and Precautions: Hawthorn is safe for long-term use and for use during pregnancy and nursing.

5-HTP (5-HYDROXYTRYPTOPHAN) The compound 5-hydroxytryptophan, or 5-HTP, is a derivative of the African plant *Griffonia simplicifolia*. This natural supplement is effective in treating conditions in which serotonin levels are low; for example, **depression, insomnia, fibromyalgia,** and **headache and migraine.** There has also been some success in treating **obesity** with 5-HTP.

Once 5-HTP enters the body, it is converted to the neurotransmitter serotonin at a rate of about 70 percent. This excellent conversion rate makes 5-HTP equally and sometimes more effective than drugs given to raise serotonin levels, and with much less severe side effects associated with drug use. Tryptophan, which also converts to serotonin, does so at a much lower rate (about 3 percent) and is available only by prescription.

What to Buy: Tablets.

How to Use: General dosage is 50 to 300 mg, from one to three times daily, depending on the condition treated. See individual medical entries for specific dosages. 5-HTP requires adequate amounts of vitamin B_6, magnesium, and niacin to convert to serotonin.

Possible Side Effects and Precautions: Mild nausea, heartburn, flatulence, and a feeling of fullness in the abdomen are experienced by some people who take 5-HTP.

INOSITOL Inositol is a B vitamin component that the body uses to produce lecithin and to transfer fats from the liver to cells in the body. Inositol also aids in reducing high cholesterol levels (see **atherosclerosis**) and is used in the treatment of **diabetes, depression,** and **Raynaud's disease.** Food sources of inositol include dried beans, chickpeas, lentils, cantaloupe, nuts, citrus, whole-grain products, and wheat germ.

What to Buy: Tablets.

How to Use: The adequate intake for inositol is 500 to 1,000 mg.

Possible Side Effects and Precautions: Heavy consumption of caffeine can cause a deficiency of inositol.

IRON Iron is a mineral found in the hemoglobin, the part of the blood that carries oxygen from the lungs to the rest of the body. It is also found in myoglobin, a protein that fuels the muscles during exercise. Iron deficiency leaves the body's tissues lacking in sufficient oxygen, which can result in iron-deficient **anemia** and fatigue.

The DRI for iron is 10 mg for adult men and women, although premenopausal women need 15 mg and pregnant women need 30 mg. Dietary sources of iron come in two forms: heme iron, found in animal sources such as chicken, red meat, and seafood; and nonheme iron, found in whole grains, nuts, dried fruit, dark green vegetables, and other plants. The body absorbs heme iron somewhat more easily than it does nonheme iron; however, if you eat nonheme iron along with heme iron foods or foods containing vitamin C, iron absorption greatly improves.

Iron deficiency can have many causes. For premenopausal women menstruation is the most common cause. Intake of certain foods and drugs can contribute to iron deficiency, including coffee, tea, soy-based products, tetracycline, and antacids, as well as high doses of calcium, zinc, and manganese supplements. Some people have a greater need for iron, including individuals who have hemorrhoids, bleeding stomach ulcers, Crohn's disease, or other conditions that cause poor absorption of iron or abnormal blood loss. People who take aspirin routinely, vegetarians, and long-distance runners also often need to supplement with iron. People who fall into any of the above-mentioned categories are potential candidates for iron supplementation. In addition, physicians may prescribe iron for women with **endometriosis** or those having difficulty with **infertility.** However, experts emphasize that no one should take iron supplements without first getting an evaluation from a knowledgeable health-care practitioner as to his or her iron needs. Excess iron is toxic and causes serious side effects (see "Side Effects" below).

What to Buy: The recommended formulation includes ferrous fumarate, ferrous peptinate, and iron glycinate, in liquid or tablets. These are less likely to cause constipation and indigestion, two side effects of iron supplementation, although some individuals experience such reactions even when using these forms. Do not buy iron sulfate or iron gluconate.

How to Use: Take iron supplements only under a doctor's care. Iron is best absorbed when taken thirty minutes before a meal.

Side Effects and Precautions: Excessive intake of iron—whether the result of megadosing or from taking iron when you do not have a deficiency—can inhibit function of the immune system, interfere with the absorption of phosphorus; cause headache, constipation, fatigue, dizziness, and vomiting; damage the intestinal tract; and increase the risk of cirrhosis, cancer, and heart attack. Taking too much iron can be a problem for the 1 out of every 250 Americans who has a genetic condition called hemochromatosis, which causes him or her to absorb twice as much iron from food and supplements as other people do. The excess iron, which is stored in the brain, heart, liver, and pancreas, usually does not cause significant damage until after age fifty.

Interactions: Iron absorption increases when it is taken with vitamin C or vitamin A and is decreased by intake of caffeine, calcium, and high-fiber foods.

LECITHIN Lecithin is a natural compound that is required by every cell in the body. It is the primary ingredient in cell membranes; without it the membranes would harden and the cells would die. Lecithin also is in the protective coverings of the brain and muscle and nerve cells. These important functions of lecithin make it a critical nutrient in the prevention of **gallstones** and **heart problems.** Its healing qualities have made it the target of studies in the prevention of **Alzheimer's disease, Parkinson's disease,** and other disorders characterized by involuntary muscle movement. Lecithin also enhances brain function, increases energy levels, and aids in the digestion of fats. Lecithin works by preventing the buildup of cholesterol and other fats in the blood vessels and vital organs and eliminating them from the body. Lecithin is also frequently used to treat **acne, chronic fatigue syndrome, fibrocystic breast disease, glaucoma, menopause,** and **Raynaud's disease.**

Many people are confused by the difference among lecithin, choline, and phosphatidylcholine. To scientists and doctors "lecithin" is the same as phosphatidylcholine, yet the general population and supplement manufacturers use the term when referring to supplements that contain phosphatidylcholine as well as other ingredients. Often the suggested supplements listed for a specific condition will indicate that either lecithin or choline, for example, is effective. Refer to the condition you wish to treat in Part II to see which form is most appropriate.

Lecithin contains various elements, including choline

(one of the B vitamins), phosphorus, inositol, and fatty acids. Dietary sources of lecithin include soybeans, lentils, green beans, chickpeas, cauliflower, corn, eggs, and wheat germ. Choline is available as a separate supplement; however, it can make those who take it smell like fish, so a lecithin supplement is preferred. Lecithin supplements are generally not needed by anyone who eats a well-balanced diet.

What to Buy: The preferred form is unbleached lecithin made from soybeans (soya) and available as granules, gel caps (usually 1,200 mg), and liquid. Most lecithin is made of soybeans; egg lecithin, derived from egg yolks, is also available. The guideline for buying a lecithin supplement is to check the ratio of lecithin/phosphatidylcholine/choline, which should be approximately 50:10:1.

How to Use: To obtain the 300 to 1,000 mg daily of choline suggested for adults, take 5 to 10 g or 1 to 2 Tbs granules that are 20 percent phosphatidylcholine; or 1,100 to 2,200 mg of 90 percent phosphatidylcholine.

Possible Side Effects and Precautions: If nausea, vomiting, bloating, abdominal pain, dizziness, or diarrhea occur, discontinue use and contact your physician. Lecithin unites with iron, iodine, and calcium to enhance brain function.

LICORICE Licorice (*Glycyrrhiza glabra*) is a sweet herb that is useful both for its medicinal qualities and as an ingredient in herbal formulas to mask any unpleasant tastes. It is a major herb in Chinese medicine, where it is used to treat conditions of the digestive and urinary tract. Among Western peoples it is most commonly used to treat **AIDS, allergies/asthma, canker sores, constipation, eczema, heartburn, herpes, PMS, ulcers, liver problems** such as hepatitis and cirrhosis, and cough and sore throat.

The active ingredients in licorice include glycyrrhizin and flavonoids. Glycyrrhizin is an antiinflammatory and antiviral substance, while the flavonoids are potent antioxidants, which help protect liver cells. Licorice acts as a mild laxative and also provides a protective coating to the stomach, which helps prevent stomach ulcers. When used for digestive disorders, a form of licorice called deglycyrrhizinated licorice, or DGL, is preferred, because the glycyrrhizin causes an increase in blood pressure in many people (see below).

What to Buy: The recommended forms are dry powdered extract, fluid extract, and powdered root in capsules. Licorice is also available in chewable tablets, dried root, and lotion. Deglycyrrhizinated licorice is preferred for most cases, as glycyrrhizin causes side effects (see below). Regular licorice, with glycyrrhizin, is indicated for respiratory infections and herpes.

How to Use: General dosages, taken up to three times daily, include 1 to 2 g powdered root capsules, 2 to 4 mL fluid extract, or 250 to 500 mg dry powdered extract. See individual medical entries for specific dosages.

Possible Side Effects and Precautions: Mild cases of upset stomach, diarrhea, headache, edema, and grogginess may occur when taking either form of licorice. An increase in blood pressure and edema may occur in people who are susceptible to glycyrrhizin. This effect is usually seen in people who take more than 1 g of glycyrrhizin daily for more than several weeks; therefore a DGL form is preferred. Avoid licorice if you have kidney failure, a history of high blood pressure, or if you take medication for heart problems. Consult your physician before starting licorice.

MAGNESIUM Magnesium is an important mineral for the formation of bone, proteins, cells, and fatty acids. It also stimulates activity of B vitamins, assists in clotting of blood, relaxes the muscles, aids in metabolism of carbohydrates and minerals, and helps form ATP (adenosine triphosphate), the fuel on which the body runs.

Although magnesium is in many foods, including nuts, grains, dark green vegetables, brown rice, garlic, apples, bananas, beans, dairy products, and fish, many people have a deficiency. Symptoms of a magnesium deficiency are fatigue, muscle weakness, depression, abnormal heart rhythms, and loss of appetite. People who are most likely to be magnesium deficient are those who take laxatives or potassium-depleting drugs, or individuals with diabetes, heart failure, or an alcohol abuse problem.

Magnesium supplementation may be helpful for people who have **allergies, backache, chronic fatigue syndrome, diabetes, heart problems, fibromyalgia, glaucoma,** high cholesterol (see **atherosclerosis**), **headache and migraine, hemorrhoids, high blood pressure, kidney stones, osteoarthritis, osteoporosis, Parkinson's disease,** and **PMS.**

What to Buy: Because magnesium can compete with other minerals for absorption, it is best to get your magnesium in a multivitamin-mineral supplement and/or with your calcium supplement.

How to Use: Dosage depends on the indication and the amount of calcium also taken. A 2:1 ratio of calcium to magnesium is recommended by many physicians, although some suggest a 1:1 dosage ratio. Michael Murray, ND, recommends basing intake on body weight: 6 mg per 2.2 pounds body weight. For example, a 110-pound woman would take 300 mg as a dietary supplement. If she had a specific medical condition to treat, the recommendation is for 12 mg per 2.2 pounds body weight.

Magnesium works closely with calcium and with vitamin B$_6$ and should be taken with these nutrients.

Possible Side Effects and Precautions: Excessive magnesium, which can mean as little as 350 to 500 mg for some people, can cause diarrhea. People who have kidney disease should avoid magnesium supplements.

MANGANESE Manganese is a mineral essential for healthy bone, skin, connective tissue, nerves, and cartilage, and for the activation of the important antioxidant enzyme superoxide dismutase (SOD). It also assists in blood clotting, the production of energy from food, and in the synthesis of protein. Good dietary sources include nuts, wheat bran, leafy green vegetables, pineapple, and seeds.

The estimated minimum daily requirement for manganese is 2.5 to 5 mg, and most people do not consume enough to fall within that range. However, serious deficiencies are rare. People with **osteoporosis** usually have low blood levels of manganese and can benefit from supplementation, as can people with **backache, diabetes, rheumatoid arthritis,** or those who have damaged their ligaments or tendons. Low levels of manganese have also been linked with **ear infections.**

What to Buy: A multivitamin-mineral supplement that contains manganese is sufficient for most individuals. If you need a supplement, look for manganese citrate tablets or capsules.

How to Use: Take 5 to 15 mg manganese, either as part of a high-quality multivitamin-mineral combination or as individual capsules or tablets. Take with meals.

Possible Side Effects and Precautions: Manganese is very safe at the levels found in supplements. People with cirrhosis should avoid manganese supplements because they may not be able to properly excrete this mineral.

Interactions: Manganese works with copper and zinc to activate SOD. Both calcium and iron reduce the amount of manganese the body can absorb.

MELATONIN Melatonin is a natural hormone that controls the body's internal clock. It is produced at night and secreted by the pineal gland, which is located deep within the brain. Levels of melatonin in the body fluctuate within a twenty-four-hour period, with the peak at night during production and the lowest levels during daylight hours. Aging also has an effect on melatonin levels, as the amount of the hormone in the body decreases with age.

Melatonin levels are typically low in people who have **insomnia** and in the elderly, which is why these populations have trouble sleeping. People who work night shifts, travel frequently across time zones, or otherwise experience jet lag can benefit from taking melatonin, as it readjusts sleep patterns. There is also some evidence that melatonin may help prevent **cataracts.**

What to Buy: Look for the time-release capsules or tablets, typically available in 750-mcg and 3-mg strengths.

How to Use: Do not take melatonin during the day. Take 1 to 3 mg one to two hours before retiring. Elderly individuals may need to take a higher dose.

Possible Side Effects and Precautions: Some people experience morning grogginess, headache, upset stomach, dizziness, disorientation, and sleepwalking. People who are pregnant or nursing or who suffer with depression, schizophrenia, kidney disease, or an autoimmune disease should not take melatonin. Melatonin can affect levels of growth hormone; therefore, it should not be taken by anyone younger than age twenty. For optimal effectiveness, keep melatonin in the refrigerator.

MILK THISTLE Milk thistle (*Silybum marianum*) has been used for more than two thousand years to treat **liver problems,** such as cirrhosis and hepatitis, and **gallstones.** The medicinal part of the plant is the seeds of the dried flower, which contains silymarin. This bioflavonoid stimulates the liver to produce healthy liver cells and acts as an antioxidant to protect the liver from damage from free radicals. Milk thistle is also helpful in the treatment of **psoriasis.**

What to Buy: Two forms are effective: the extract, standardized to 70 to 80 percent silymarin; and the extract with silymarin bound to phosphatidylcholine (a component of cell membranes). Both can be found in capsules and as a tincture. Milk thistle is also available as dry bulk seeds.

How to Use: The standard dosage for extract standardized to 70 to 80 percent silymarin is 70 to 210 mg three times daily. For extracts with phosphatidylcholine-bound silymarin 100 to 200 mg twice daily is the usual dosage. The tincture can be taken at 10 to 25 drops up to three times daily. The dried, powdered seeds can be made into an infusion (2 to 3 tsp steeped in 8 oz hot water for ten to fifteen minutes) or added to food; 1 tsp three times daily. See individual medical entries for specific dosages.

Possible Side Effects and Precautions: Milk thistle is considered very safe, even for women who are pregnant or lactating. It may cause loose stools in some people, but this effect usually disappears in two to three days.

MYRRH Myrrh (*Commiphora molmol*) was a common remedy among ancient peoples for treatment of infections, dental problems, and bad breath. Today those uses have not changed much: myrrh is taken for **canker sores, common cold and flu,** and **gingivitis.** It is effective because it stimulates production of white blood cells and has strong antibacterial activity.

Myrrh is an oil found in the bark of several different African and Arabian shrubs. The oil hardens into a resin, which is dried and powdered for use.

What to Buy: The preferred forms are tincture, powder, or capsule, depending on the use. Myrrh is also found in some tooth products.

How to Use: To make a tea, steep 1 to 2 tsp powdered

herb in 8 oz boiling water for ten to fifteen minutes. Drink three times daily. To make a mouthwash, steep 1 tsp powdered herb and 1 tsp boric acid in 16 oz boiling water. Let stand thirty minutes, strain, and use when cool. Other general dosages include 1 capsule three times daily and 1 to 2 mL tincture three times daily.

Possible Side Effects and Precautions: Mild stomach upset and diarrhea may occur. If myrrh is taken in large doses, it can cause vomiting, nausea, sweating, kidney problems, and heart palpitations. Do not take if you are pregnant, nursing, or have kidney disease.

NETTLE Nettle, or stinging nettle (*Urtica dioica*), gets its name from the fact that the tiny hairs on the leaves sting or burn when they touch the skin. When the plant is dried, however, it loses its stinging abilities. The medicinal parts of the plant include the root and leaves, which traditionally have been used to treat coughs, arthritis, and tuberculosis. Today nettle is used to treat hay fever (see **allergies**), **urinary-tract infections,** and benign prostatic hyperplasia (see **prostate problems**).

The active substances in nettle are believed to be lectins (protein-sugar molecules) and polysaccharides (complex sugars). Nettle leaves prevent the body from producing prostaglandins, which cause inflammation, and the roots affect the sex hormones.

What to Buy: The preferred forms are capsules, root extract, and dried root for decoctions. Also available are tablets, tincture, and dried whole herb.

How to Use: See individual medical entries for specific dosages. To prepare a decoction, steep 1 tsp dried root in 8 oz hot water and divide into two doses for the day.

Possible Side Effects and Precautions: No side effects have been noted.

NIACIN AND NIACINAMIDE (VITAMIN B₃) Niacin and niacinamide are the two main forms of vitamin B_3. Both substances are key in helping release energy from carbohydrates, processing alcohol, and forming fats. A significant benefit of niacin is its ability to prevent recurrent heart attack. Niacin also helps regulate cholesterol levels. A third form of niacin, inositol hexaniacinate, is gaining acceptance as a substitute for niacin. Inositol hexaniacinate is composed of one molecule of inositol (an "unofficial" B vitamin) and six molecules of niacin. (See the entry for **inositol** for more details.)

Vitamin B_3 is found in high levels in peanuts, brewer's yeast, and fish, and in lesser amounts in whole grains. Signs of deficiency include rash, diarrhea, emotional and mental changes, loss of appetite, an inflamed tongue, and digestive problems. Niacin deficiency is rare in Western cultures, largely because niacin is added to white flour, and Americans consume a great deal of products made from white flour.

Many people have a negative reaction to niacin supplements (see "Possible Side Effects and Precautions" p. 64). Niacinamide and inositol are safe alternatives, but they do not have the heart-protective advantages provided by niacin. Niacin and niacinamide supplements are used to treat **depression,** high cholesterol (see **atherosclerosis**), **insomnia, osteoarthritis, rheumatoid arthritis,** and **Raynaud's disease.**

What to Buy: A multivitamin-mineral or a B-complex supplement that contains niacin and/or niacinamide is sufficient for most individuals. Both forms of vitamin B_3 are available individually as tablets and capsules. Niacinamide is preferred by many individuals because it does not cause the side effects associated with niacin (see "Possible Side Effects" p. 64). If you prefer to take niacin or your physician has approved it for you, do not buy sustained-release or slow-release niacin products, because they can be very harmful to the liver.

How to Use: To lower cholesterol (see **atherosclerosis**) large doses of niacin are needed. Strict supervision by a physician is necessary, however, because liver damage is possible. For **osteoarthritis** high levels of niacinamide are recommended, depending on the severity of the disease. At least three months of treatment are needed for results to become apparent, and continued use is required for relief. To treat depression niacin plus niacinamide and **inositol** are recommended. Take niacin with food to reduce the chance of stomach upset.

Possible Side Effects and Precautions: Flushing, a feeling of heat on the face and sometimes the entire body, nausea, and itching are associated with niacin. These side effects are temporary, lasting several minutes to about one hour. More serious effects include dark urine, yellow skin or eyes, and loss of appetite. If you have liver disease or low blood pressure, do not take niacin. Use of niacin or niacinamide may cause any of the following conditions to become worse: diabetes, glaucoma, gout, bleeding disorders, or stomach ulcer.

Interactions: Niacin can decrease the effectiveness of insulin in diabetics and increase the effects of antihypertensive drugs in people with high blood pressure.

OATS Oats (*Avena ativa*) are a widely used supplement for treatment of skin disorders such as **eczema** and **shingles.** The oats used in supplements are derived from wild species that are now cultivated worldwide, and they come in a variety of forms (see "What to Buy," p. 65). Several parts of the plant are used medicinally. The seeds contain alkaloids, iron, manganese, and zinc; the straw has a high silica content. Alkaloids in the plant are believed to be responsible for the plant's ability to soothe and heal.

What to Buy: The recommended form for treatment of skin disorders is the dried herb, sometimes referred to as oat straw.

How to Use: See **eczema** and **shingles** for instructions on how to use oats in the bath.

Possible Side Effects and Precautions: No known side effects noted when oats are used externally.

OMEGA-3 FATTY ACIDS Omega-3 fatty acids are perhaps best known for their ability to help prevent heart disease by lowering the blood level of low-density lipoprotein (LDL), which is the harmful type of cholesterol that leads to **atherosclerosis.** Supplementation with omega-3 fatty acids also helps enhance blood circulation, relieves inflammation associated with **osteoarthritis** and **inflammatory bowel disease** (colitis), relieves skin problems such as **psoriasis,** and helps thin the blood.

Omega-3 fatty acids are versatile fatty molecules found in certain fish (cold-water fish such as sardines, mackerel, and tuna), walnuts, and canola oil. The world's richest source, however, is flaxseed oil. There are two types of omega-3's—EPA, eicosapentaenoic acid, and DHA, docosahexaenoic acid. These fatty acids keep the cell membranes pliable so the cells can pass easily through blood vessels and suppress the production of leukotrienes, substances that cause inflammation. Both fish oils and flaxseed oil supply EPA and DHA, although flaxseed oil provides a lesser amount of EPA. However, flaxseed oil does not cause the side effects associated with fish oil—namely, increases in blood sugar and LDL cholesterol levels, nosebleeds, gastrointestinal problems, and a burping "fishy" smell.

Often inflammation is caused by too much of another omega fatty acid—omega-6, which is found in evening primrose oil and several other plants. Maintaining a proper balance of these two fatty acids is important to help prevent pain related to inflammation (see **evening primrose oil**). Flaxseed oil contains a balance of these two fatty acids.

What to Buy: Flaxseed oil is the preferred source of omega-3 fatty acid and contains more than twice the amount of omega-3 found in fish oils. Look for organic, unrefined flaxseed oil, available either as oil or in capsules.

How to Use: Flaxseed oil can be used in salads or on vegetables. Do not use it for cooking. One tablespoon, or five capsules, daily is the suggested supplement dosage.

Possible Side Effects and Precautions: Fish oil can cause blood sugar levels and LDL cholesterol levels to rise. Nose-bleeds can occur because fish oil thins the blood, and gastrointestinal problems, along with burping "fishy" smells, affect some people. People with heart disease or diabetes should consult with their physician before taking fish oil. Flaxseed oil does not cause side effects.

Interactions: Because fish oil is easily damaged by oxygen (oxidation), take only fish-oil supplements that contain at least a few milligrams or IUs of vitamin E. An additional vitamin E supplement of 200 IU is also recommended. Fish oil can increase the anticoagulant effects of anticoagulant medications, including aspirin. Consult with your physician before starting any omega-3 supplements.

PANTOTHENIC ACID (VITAMIN B_5) Pantothenic acid, or vitamin B_5, is part of the vitamin B complex. It has several critical roles in the body, including helping to convert proteins, carbohydrates, and fats into energy and aiding in the production of hormones and antibodies. It is referred to as an "antistress" vitamin by many experts because of its ability to relieve **depression** and anxiety. Pantothenic acid is also helpful in treating **gout** and gynecological problems. Pantothenic acid works synergistically with vitamins B_1, B_2, and B_3 to make fuel for the body in the form of ATP.

Pantothenic acid can be found in all foods (*pantothenic* is derived from a Greek word that means "from every-where"). The best sources include brewer's yeast, wheat germ, wheat bran, peanuts, peas, whole grains, broccoli, mushrooms, and sweet potatoes. Deficiency is rare, although people who abuse alcohol are likely to have low levels and are the best candidates for supplementation.

What to Buy: A multivitamin-mineral supplement that contains either d-calcium pantothenate or pantothenic acid is adequate for many people. For additional amounts pantothenic acid is available in capsules and tablets and in extended-release form.

How to Use: If you take pantothenic acid as a separate supplement, take it along with a **B complex.**

Possible Side Effects and Precautions: Pantothenic acid is safe at suggested supplemental doses but may cause diarrhea if you take several grams per day.

PEPPERMINT Peppermint (*Mentha piperita*) is actually a hybrid of two other mints—spearmint and water mint—and was first cultivated in 1750. Several different forms of peppermint are grown, and all are effective in the treatment of **nausea/morning sickness,** and menstrual problems.

Since it was first recognized for its healing powers, peppermint has been used to treat stomach and intestinal problems, including **irritable bowel syndrome.** Today it is also used to relieve **heartburn, gallstones,** and **nausea/ morning sickness.** The pure volatile oils, which contain menthol alone and menthol combined with other substances, appear to be the compounds that provide pain relief. They may also help tone the digestive system and promote the flow of bile from the gallbladder.

What to Buy: The preferred forms are dried leaves (for infusions), enteric-coated capsules (oil), and tincture. Also available as tablets.

How to Use: To prepare an infusion, use 1 to 2 heaping

tsp per 8 oz boiling water and steep for ten minutes. Drink up to 3 cups daily. The suggested dosage for capsules is 2 or 3 daily between meals. See individual medical entries for specific dosages.

Possible Side Effects and Precautions: Do not ingest pure peppermint oil or pure menthol, as both are very toxic and, in the case of menthol, can be fatal. Those who should avoid using peppermint include women with a history of miscarriage and anyone with gallbladder or bile-duct inflammation, obstruction, or a related condition.

PHOSPHORUS Phosphorus is the second most abundant mineral in the body (calcium is the first), with 85 percent of it found in the bones and teeth. As the two most common minerals in the body, calcium and phosphorus depend on each other and must maintain a stable ratio (1:2 is ideal) to keep the body healthy. Another indication of the close relationship between calcium and phosphorus is that the RDA for phosphorus is similar to that for calcium: 800 mg for adults and 1,200 mg for pregnant or nursing women.

Phosphorus is found in all cells and is a key factor in the growth and maintenance of cells and tissues and in energy production. Few people have a deficiency of phosphorus; in fact, many people actually consume too much phosphorus, given that one serving of most soft drinks supplies up to 500 mg and that many convenience foods contain phosphoric acid as a preservative. Excessive levels of phosphorus contribute to a loss of calcium, especially from bone, which can lead to **osteoporosis.** Phosphorus is also found in many different foods, including meat and dairy products, nuts, beans, and grains, with lesser amounts in vegetables and fruits.

Individuals most likely to be deficient in phosphorus are those who take large amounts of aluminum-containing antacids, and people who have kidney or liver disorders, any condition that hinders metabolism of vitamin D, or alcoholism. Signs of deficiency are fatigue, loss of appetite, weakness, bone pain, reduced bone mineralization, and muscle tremors.

What to Buy: Most people have no need to take phosphorus supplements. If you do, they are available in tablets and capsules.

How to Use: Phosphorus supplements should be taken only under supervision of your physician and as part of a well-balanced supplement plan.

Possible Side Effects and Precautions: Although phosphorus supplements are not known to cause side effects, an excessive amount of this mineral can damage calcium metabolism and absorption.

POTASSIUM Potassium is a mineral needed to maintain a regular heart rhythm, blood pressure, neuromuscular functioning, acid levels, and water balance. Levels of potassium tend to be low in people who are taking diuretics ("water pills") or laxatives or who have chronic diarrhea or kidney disorders. Potassium works closely with sodium to regulate blood pressure, water levels, muscle tone, and other functions. Good food sources of potassium include fruit, especially bananas, apricots, and figs; also beans, garlic, brown rice, nuts, potatoes, raisins, winter squash, and yams.

Potassium is helpful for individuals who have congestive heart failure or **high blood pressure.** However, dietary potassium is preferred over supplements, because the latter often cause side effects (see "Possible Side Effects," p. 70). Studies show that a diet low in potassium and high in sodium (salt) increases the risk of heart disease, stroke, and high blood pressure. This imbalance is particularly critical if you have kidney disease or high blood pressure or if you are taking certain medications, such as ACE inhibitors or potassium-sparing drugs.

What to Buy: Over-the-counter potassium is available in 99-mg tablets, timed-release tablets, effervescent tablets, and capsules; it is also dispensed by prescription. Potassium supplements are sold as potassium salts (chloride and bicarbonate) or potassium bound to different mineral chelates (e.g., aspartate, citrate).

How to Use: One 99-mg tablet or capsule daily for people who have heart problems. Potassium supplements should be taken under supervision of a physician.

Possible Side Effects and Precautions: Potassium supplements can irritate the stomach if taken in amounts greater than 99 mg. The potassium available in fruit (a banana has 500 mg, for example) does not cause this side effect.

PSYLLIUM Psyllium is a flowering herb that produces small brown seed pods, which have been used for centuries to treat **constipation, diarrhea, diverticulitis, gallstones,** and **hemorrhoids.**It is still used to treat all of these conditions, as well as **ulcers** and colitis.

Psyllium seeds are a rich source of fiber, which is the ingredient that makes this herb so effective. It is also the reason many commercial laxatives contain psyllium as their main ingredient.

What to Buy: Whole, ground, or powdered seeds; also husks. Psyllium is also found in many commercial bulk-forming laxative products.

How to Use: If you have been eating a low-fiber diet, begin gradually with 1/2 tsp psyllium seeds or powder mixed in 8 oz cool liquid and drink 2 to 3 cups daily. Increase to 1 tsp per 8 oz after one or two days. Stir the mixture vigorously and drink it quickly, followed by additional water. When taking psyllium it is important to drink at least eight to ten additional glasses of water daily to prevent blockage of the intestinal tract.

Possible Side Effects and Precautions: People who are allergic to grasses or dust may have an allergic reaction to psyllium. Severe reactions are rare. Do not use psyllium if you are pregnant, because it can stimulate the lower pelvis.

PYRIDOXINE (VITAMIN B₆) Pyridoxine, or vitamin B_6, is one of the water-soluble B-complex vitamins. Its main functions in the body are to help release energy from food (metabolism), aid in the proper functioning of more than sixty enzymes, promote a healthy immune system, help in cell multiplication, and assist in the manufacture of genetic material called nucleic acid.

Large concentrations of pyridoxine are found in the brain. This has led to its use in treating **depression.** It is also used to treat **acne, allergies, carpal tunnel syndrome, diabetes, ear infections, endometriosis, fibrocystic breast disease, headache, insomnia, kidney stones, multiple sclerosis, nausea, Parkinson's disease, PMS, prostate problems,** and **seborrheic dermatitis.**

Natural sources of pyridoxine include brown rice, bananas, avocados, whole grains, lentils, corn, liver, and nuts. A deficiency of pyridoxine usually occurs with other deficiencies in the B complex and manifests with symptoms such as weakness, inflamed tongue and mouth, sleeplessness, and nerve problems in the feet and hands.

What to Buy: Look for pyridoxine available as pyridoxal-5-phosphate, which is more bioavailable than the other form, pyridoxine hydrochloride. Both forms are sold as tablets and capsules and in extended-release formulas. The pyridoxine hydrochloride form is sufficient as long as you get enough riboflavin and magnesium in your diet or in supplements.

How to Use: The most common supplement dosage is 10 to 25 mg, but a physician may recommend 200 mg or more depending on your needs. Do not crush or chew the capsules or tablets. Pyridoxine increases the bioavailability of magnesium, so it is suggested that you take these nutrients together. See individual medical entries for specific dosages.

Possible Side Effects and Precautions: If taken in excessive amounts (200 mg or more per day) for a long period of time, pyridoxine may cause loss of sensation in the hands and feet and difficulty walking. If you are taking the drug levodopa, consult with your physician before taking pyridoxine.

QUERCETIN Quercetin belongs to a group of nutrients known as bioflavonoids (or flavonoids), which are water-soluble plant pigments. It is a powerful antioxidant, antihistamine, and antiinflammatory agent, which makes it useful in the prevention and treatment of **atherosclerosis, bronchitis, colds and flu, cataracts, gingivitis,** and hay fever (see **allergies**). In the treatment of allergies and **eczema,** for example, quercetin prohibits the release of histamine, which causes allergic reactions.

The best food sources of quercetin are apples, black tea, citrus fruit, and onions, with lesser amounts found in leafy green vegetables and beans.

What to Buy: Quercetin is derived from blue-green algae and is available as a single nutrient or in combination with other bioflavonoids (e.g., rutin, hesperidin) and/or with vitamin C and occasionally with herbs that are rich in bioflavonoids (e.g., ginkgo). Look for tablets and capsules in 200-, 500-, and 1,000-mg doses.

How to Use: Generally suggested dosage is 400 mg two to three times daily. Quercetin and other bioflavonoids enhance the absorption of vitamin C, so they should be taken together.

Possible Side Effects and Precautions: Quercetin can cause diarrhea if taken in extremely high doses (more than 5,000 mg daily).

RIBOFLAVIN (VITAMIN B₂) Riboflavin, or vitamin B_2, is part of the complex of water-soluble B vitamins. It plays a primary role in processing amino acids and fats, forming red blood cells, converting carbohydrates into energy, activating vitamin B_6 and folic acid, and maintaining the mucous membranes in the digestive tract. Supplementation with riboflavin can be effective in the prevention and treatment of **cataracts.**

Good food sources include beans, soybean products, eggs, spinach, yogurt, and meat. People who have an increased need for riboflavin include women who take oral contraceptives and anyone who participates in routine strenuous activity. Signs that you may be deficient in riboflavin include sores and cracks at the corners of the mouth; oily, dry, scaly skin; sensitivity to light; and swollen, red, painful tongue. Pregnant women need to be particularly careful to consume enough riboflavin, because a deficiency can cause damage to the fetus.

What to Buy: The amount of riboflavin in good-quality multivitamin-mineral supplements or B-complex supplements is sufficient for most people. Look on the label for activated riboflavin (riboflav-5-phosphate) or simply riboflavin. Also available as a sole nutrient in tablet form.

How to Use: Take with food to improve absorption.

Possible Side Effects and Precautions: Riboflavin may cause the urine to turn a dark yellow, but this is a completely harmless side effect.

ST. JOHN'S WORT St. John's wort (*Hypericum perforatum*) is a flowering herb that is taken internally to treat mild to moderate **depression** and applied externally to heal burns, cuts, and abrasions. Its yellow flowers contain the active ingredient hypericin, which has antidepressant, antiinflammatory, and antibacterial properties. Flavonoids have also been identified in the flowers, and this finding leads researchers to suggests St. John's wort also may boost the immune system. Its ability to stop certain viruses from reproducing suggests St. John's wort has the potential to treat AIDS, although more research is needed. It is sometimes used to treat **fibromyalgia.**

What to Buy: Look for a standardized hypericin content of 0.3 percent in capsules, tincture, and extract. Also available as dried leaves and flowers (containing 0.2 to 1.0 percent hypericin) to make infusions and as an ointment for topical use.

How to Use: St. John's wort should be taken with meals to avoid gastric upset. The average tincture dosage is 15 to 40 drops up to three times daily. To prepare an infusion from the dried leaves and flowers, add 1 to 2 tsp dried herb to 8 oz boiling water. Cover and allow to steep for fifteen minutes. Drink up to 3 cups daily. Follow application directions on commercial ointment products. Crushed flowers and leaves can be applied to cleaned wounds.

Possible Side Effects and Precautions: St. John's wort should be taken under a doctor's supervision. In a few people this herb can cause high blood pressure, headache, stiff neck, nausea, vomiting, and sensitivity to light (photosensitivity).

Interactions: St. John's wort may interact with the amino acids tryptophan and tyrosine; amphetamines; diet pills; nasal decongestants; beverages such as beer, wine, and coffee; foods such as chocolate, fava beans, smoked or pickled foods, yogurt, and salami; and cold or allergy medications. The most common reactions include nausea and high blood pressure.

SAW PALMETTO Saw palmetto (*Serenoa repens*) is a shrub which bears berries that are used to treat a common problem among men, benign enlargement of the prostate gland (see **prostate problems**). Saw palmetto is effective because it apparently blocks production of the chemical dihydrotestosterone, which is believed to cause this prostate problem. Urinary flow, which is often significantly reduced in men with prostate problems, can improve by 50 percent or more in men who take saw palmetto. Other conditions that may respond to this herb include respiratory disorders and nasal congestion.

What to Buy: The most effective form is the extract standardized to contain 85 to 95 percent fatty acids and sterols. Although nonstandardized tinctures, fluid extracts, and crude berries are available, they are not as effective.

How to Use: The recommended dosage of standardized extract is 160 mg twice daily.

Possible Side Effects and Precautions: No side effects have been noted.

SELENIUM Selenium is a trace mineral that is believed to be a potent protector against **cancer.** This belief comes from selenium's ability to activate the very powerful antioxidant enzyme glutathione peroxidase. Selenium also stimulates the thyroid hormones, prevents buildup of fats in the blood vessels, enhances immune-system functioning, and protects against heavy-metal poisoning.

It's been shown in more than twenty countries that the lower the intake of selenium, the higher the incidence of cancer of the colon, breast, pancreas, ovary, bladder, prostate, rectum, skin, and lungs. Other conditions that may respond to supplementation with selenium include **AIDS, allergies, atherosclerosis, cataracts, macular degeneration, multiple sclerosis,** and **rheumatoid arthritis.**

Natural sources include whole grains, asparagus, garlic, and mushrooms.

What to Buy: Look for capsules and softgels, the latter

of which are usually in combination with vitamin E. Some nutritionists say that a natural form of selenium, called L-selenomethionine or selenium-rich yeast, is superior to synthetic forms. This has not been proven.

How to Use: Typical supplemental dosage is 200 mcg daily. Do not take higher doses unless you are under a doctor's care.

Possible Side Effects and Precautions: Taking excessive amounts of selenium (1,000 mcg or more) can cause rash, changes in the nervous system, and loss of fingernails.

SKULLCAP Skullcap (*Scutellaria baicalensis, S. lateriflora*) is a Chinese herb that has gained acceptance among Westerners, especially as a safe treatment for **insomnia.** Since it was first mentioned in Chinese writings back in A.D. 250–330, it has been valued as a diuretic, an antiinflammatory, and for its calming effect. Today it is used for a variety of conditions, including nervous tension, tension **headache,** and alcohol withdrawal.

What to Buy: The preferred forms are capsules, tincture, and dried leaves for infusions. Also available are tablets and the prepared tea.

How to Use: The average dosage for the tincture is 20 to 40 drops up to four times daily; for the capsules, up to six 425-mg capsules per day. To prepare an infusion, pour 8 oz boiling water over 2 tsp dried herb and steep covered for ten to fifteen minutes. Drink up to 3 cups daily. Skullcap is best taken after meals.

Possible Side Effects and Precautions: Skullcap may cause drowsiness, so do not drive a car or heavy machinery after taking it. Other temporary side effects include stomach upset and diarrhea.

SULFUR (MSM) Sulfur is a mineral used by the body to manufacture the bile it needs for digestion. It is found in all the body's tissues, especially those with a high percentage of protein. The three amino acids that contain the most sulfur are cystine, cysteine, and methionine. Sulfur also is a major component of a substance called keratin, which is found in skin, hair, and nails. If you have ever smelled burning hair, the odor you smell is sulfur.

The bioavailable form of sulfur is called MSM, short for methylsulfonylmethane, which is found naturally in legumes, whole grains, vegetables, meat, and dairy. Because MSM is easily destroyed during food processing and cooking, the most reliable food sources are unprocessed, uncooked foods. Scientists have not yet determined a recommended or suggested dosage for sulfur.

The body uses MSM to build keratin and collagen, which are essential components of skin and connective tissue; and amino acids. MSM helps in the production of insulin, which leads some researchers to believe it may be beneficial for people with diabetes. Because MSM improves the ability of nutrients and waste materials to move in and out of cells and tissue more readily, it is often used to treat conditions characterized by inflammation and pain, such as **osteoarthritis** and **rheumatoid arthritis.** Other conditions that respond to MSM include **constipation** and **heartburn.**

What to Buy: Both capsules and powder are recommended for oral use; creams and sprays are for topical use.

How to Use: The powder can be dissolved in any nonalcoholic liquid or mixed with food. Creams and sprays are used for topical applications. MSM is also available in toothpastes and in eyedrops for eye infections. Earl Mindell, RPh, PhD, author of *Earl Mindell's Vitamin Bible,* suggests a daily intake of 2,000 to 6,000 mg to maintain good health. Not all experts agree. The most beneficial dosage depends on your age, body size, the level of MSM in your body before supplementation, and your overall state of health.

MSM should be taken with food to avoid possible gastrointestinal problems.

Possible Side Effects and Precautions: MSM is considered to be nontoxic at very high dosage levels—10,000 mg and more daily. However, some people experience headache and gastrointestinal problems when taking 3,000 mg or more of MSM. Proponents of MSM say these reactions indicate the body is ridding itself of toxins.

Interactions: MSM may interact with blood-thinning drugs such as aspirin, heparin, or dicumarol. If you are taking blood thinners, consult your physician before taking MSM.

TEA TREE OIL Tea tree oil is derived from the leaves of the *Melaleuca alternifolia* tree, a native of Australia. For centuries the native Australians have used the oil to treat various skin ailments. Scientific investigations show that the oil contains the active ingredient called terpineol, which is a potent antibacterial and antifungal agent. Today tea tree oil is used to prevent and treat **acne, athlete's foot, dandruff,** and other skin conditions.

What to Buy: Oil; it is also an ingredient in some health and beauty products such as toothpaste and soap.

How to Use: Apply the oil directly to the affected area.

Possible Side Effects and Precautions: If you have sensitive skin, test the oil on a small patch of skin before applying it to a wider area. To avoid getting a skin reaction, dilute the tea tree oil with vegetable oil.

THIAMIN (VITAMIN B_1) Thiamin, or vitamin B_1, is a member of the B vitamin complex. Although the body needs only a minuscule amount of thiamin, it plays several major roles in health. Thiamin assists in carbohydrate metabolism and blood formation; stimulates blood circulation; and has a part in maintaining muscle tone of the stomach, intestines, and heart.

Thiamin is found in many foods, including dried beans, oatmeal, brown rice, peanuts, peas, soybeans, wheat germ, and whole grains. A deficiency of thiamin can cause shortness of breath, low blood pressure, irregular heart rhythm, and chest pain. Low thiamin levels can also cause beriberi, a nervous-system disorder in which people experience fatigue, weight loss, gastrointestinal disorders, weakness, and tender, atrophied muscles. A thiamin deficiency can be caused by alcohol abuse and lead to significant memory impairment, problems with motor and eye movements, and poor reality perception. Other people who may have an increased need for thiamin include pregnant women and individuals who perform strenuous physical labor or activities. Certain medications, such as antibiotics, oral contraceptives, and sulfa drugs, can decrease thiamin levels in the body. When thiamin is taken as a supplement it is usually to prevent a deficiency or to treat impaired mental function in the elderly or people with **Alzheimer's disease.**

What to Buy: A high-quality multivitamin-mineral supplement should contain sufficient thiamin, usually as thiamin hydrochloride. Also available as an individual nutrient in tablet and capsule form.

How to Use: You may get the dosage you need from a vitamin B–complex supplement, or take a thiamin supplement along with a B complex.

Possible Side Effects and Precautions: Thiamin is safe when taken as directed. A dosage as low as 5 mg very rarely can cause side effects, including itching, nervousness, flushing, and an abnormally rapid heartbeat (tachycardia) in sensitive individuals. Dilantin (an epileptic drug), alcohol, and other drugs may inhibit thiamin activity.

UVA URSI From the leaves of the uva ursi (*Arctostaphylos uva-ursi*) shrub comes a substance that has been used to treat **urinary-tract problems** for at least one thousand years.

Uva ursi, also known as bearberry, contains arbutin, which converts to hydroquinone in the urinary tract. It is the hydroquinone that eliminates the infectious agents in the urinary system. It is reportedly especially effective against *E. coli.*

Uva ursi also is applied topically to treat minor skin problems, such as cuts and abrasions, to speed up tissue healing. Some evidence suggests it also has diuretic properties.

What to Buy: The recommended forms are capsules and tincture (50 percent alcohol). Also available as dried leaves and tablets.

How to Use: To make an infusion from the dried leaves, simmer 1 to 2 tsp dried leaves in 8 oz water for five to ten minutes. Drink up to 3 cups daily. Uva ursi requires an alkaline environment in order to be effective; therefore avoid eating acidic foods such as citrus fruit and juices, vitamin C, and sauerkraut during the course of taking this herb. You can take 2 tsp baking soda in a glass of water each day while taking uva ursi to help maintain an alkaline environment.

Possible Side Effects and Precautions: Because uva ursi contains a high level of tannins, it can cause nausea, vomiting, and stomach distress. Do not take this herb for longer than seven days unless you are under the guidance of a medical professional. Pregnant women should not use this herb.

VALERIAN An herb known for its calming effect is valerian (*Valeriana officinalis*). For more than one thousand years the root has been used to successfully treat **insomnia,** nervousness, tension **headache,** and menstrual cramps. It is still used for these purposes today.

Valerian is probably best known for its ability to improve the quality of sleep, hasten onset of sleep, and reduce the number of nighttime awakenings. Unlike conventional sleep aids, valerian does this without side effects, addiction, and withdrawal symptoms associated with barbiturates or benzodiazepines.

What to Buy: Look for extract standardized for at least 0.5 percent essential oil. Standardized capsules and tincture are the preferred forms. Also available as dried root for decoctions and tablets.

How to Use: For standardized capsules, take 300 to 400 mg daily. A decoction is suitable for treatment of **headache.** See individual medical entries for specific dosages.

Possible Side Effects and Precautions: Do not take valerian if you are also taking conventional tranquilizers or sedatives. Because valerian causes drowsiness, do not drive after taking it. In some individuals valerian causes excitability, mild headache, or upset stomach. In rare cases it can cause severe headache, nausea, morning grogginess, restlessness, or blurred vision.

VITAMIN A AND BETA-CAROTENE Vitamin A is a member of the antioxidant family and plays a key role in normal cell reproduction, which is necessary to prevent precancerous changes in cells. Some of its other critical functions include helping the eyes see normally in the dark, maintaining healthy cell membranes against invasion from harmful organisms, helping in the formation of bone, growth hormones, and proteins, and stimulating the immune system.

You can get vitamin A two different ways through your food. Animal-based foods (e.g., eggs, milk, liver, and fish) contain a form of vitamin A known as retinol. The vitamin A that comes from plant foods is known as carotenoids. Beta-carotene is a carotenoid that the body converts into vitamin A as it is needed. Carotenoids are found in orange, red, yellow, and dark green leafy vegetables.

Vitamin A is a fat-soluble vitamin, which means it is stored in the body. Large amounts can cause significant side effects, including headache, liver damage, bone and joint pain, abnormal bone growth, nerve damage, birth defects, and vomiting. Beta-carotene does not cause these reactions, even when it is taken in high doses. In fact, high intake of beta-carotene is beneficial, because it enhances the immune system and improves resistance to invading organisms. Generally, beta-carotene is safer and more effective than vitamin A: it does not have the significant side effects, and it has cancer- and heart-disease-prevention properties that vitamin A does not.

Both vitamin A and beta-carotene are useful in the prevention and/or treatment of **acne, bursitis, cancer, cataracts, colds and flu, constipation, ear infections** (recurrent), **eczema, gingivitis, herpes, macular degeneration, multiple sclerosis, osteoarthritis, psoriasis, seborrheic dermatitis, ulcers,** and **urinary-tract infections.** Deficiencies can occur in people who consume very limited amounts of vegetables and dairy foods. The first sign of deficiency is usually poor night vision, which may be accompanied by dry skin and an increased susceptibility to infections and problems with reproduction.

What to Buy: Beta-carotene is preferred over vitamin A, and it is recommended that you buy a high-quality multivitamin-mineral that contains beta-carotene. Some supplements state "Vitamin A (as beta-carotene)." Vitamin A used to be labeled in IUs (international units) but is now expressed in retinol equivalents (RE) to better distinguish between the two forms of vitamin A. Vitamin A is also available in capsules, tablets, and liquid; beta-carotene in capsules and tablets.

How to Use: Intake of vitamin A should be limited to less than 10,000 IU (2,000 RE) for women who are pregnant or who could become pregnant. For men and post-menopausal women, up to 25,000 IU (5,000 RE) daily is safe. The liquid form of vitamin A may be taken by drops directly into the mouth or mixed into juice or food. When taking beta–carotene, the equivalent of 25,000 IU of vitamin A activity (2,000 RE, or 6 mg) is safe, although some people take up to 100,000 IU (20,000 RE) without any problems.

Possible Side Effects and Precautions: Intake of 25,000 IU or more per day of vitamin A can cause headache, hair loss, fatigue, bone problems, dry skin, and liver damage. Beta-carotene does not cause these problems, although taking more than 100,000 IU daily can cause the skin to have a yellow-orange hue. Use of vitamin A should be limited to less than 10,000 IU daily for women who are pregnant or who could become pregnant, because there is an increased risk of birth defects.

VITAMIN B$_{12}$ Vitamin B$_{12}$, sometimes referred to as cyanocobalamin, is a key component in cell formation and longevity, proper digestion, protein synthesis, absorption of food, and metabolism of fats and carbohydrates. It also helps maintain fertility and, along with the other B vitamins, helps produce neurotransmitters, chemicals that facilitate communication between nerves. This latter function makes B$_{12}$ helpful in the prevention and treatment of **depression** and other mood disorders.

Deficiency of B$_{12}$ is nearly synonymous with **anemia**, which may be caused by inadequate consumption of B$_{12}$ or an inability to absorb it properly. Malabsorption of vitamin B$_{12}$ is common and may be caused by certain diseases, such as colitis or celiac disease, by an insufficient amount of stomach acid, abnormal bacterial growth in the intestines, or previous stomach or intestinal surgery. Supplementation with B$_{12}$ is effective for people with **allergies, atheroscle-**

rosis, backache, inflammatory bowel disease, infertility, liver problems, multiple sclerosis, and **vaginitis.**

A deficiency of B_{12} can take many years to become apparent, because the body stores this vitamin—up to 10 mg at a time—and very little is excreted. Signs of deficiency, in addition to anemia, include memory loss, abnormal gait, decreased reflexes, hallucinations, eye problems, and digestive disorders.

The best food sources of B_{12} are primarily animal products (e.g., cheese, clams, herring, liver), although many soy products and cereals are now fortified with vitamin B_{12}. Supplements are often recommended for the elderly, people with digestive disorders, and strict vegetarians.

What to Buy: Sublingual tablets are preferred, because the nutrient is readily absorbed through the mucous membranes in the mouth. B_{12} is also available in regular and extended-release tablets. Injections can be obtained from your physician.

How to Use: Treatment of specific ailments and severe deficiency often require high dosages, which may be best treated by injections from a physician. For health maintenance most high-quality multivitamin-minerals and B-complex supplements contain sufficient amounts of B_{12}. See individual medical entries for specific dosages.

Possible Side Effects and Precautions: Vitamin B_{12} can be taken at ten thousand times the DRI (2.0 to 2.6 mcg) and not cause side effects. People who take antigout or anticoagulant medications or potassium supplements may have a problem absorbing dietary B_{12} and need additional supplementation.

VITAMIN B COMPLEX A vitamin B–complex supplement contains the eight essential B vitamins in one tablet or capsule. Each of the B vitamins has its own chemical makeup, yet they perform similar functions and are found in many of the same foods. Some of the functions they share include maintaining healthy muscle and skin, enhancing the immune and nervous systems, promoting metabolism, and stimulating cell reproduction and growth. Foods rich in B vitamins include brewer's yeast, beans, peas, dark green leafy vegetables, whole-grain cereals, organ meats, and dairy products.

Because B vitamins are essential to so many functions, the complex is often recommended for a long list of conditions, including **AIDS, canker sores, carpal tunnel syndrome, cataracts, dandruff, depression, diverticulitis, eczema, endometriosis, glaucoma, gout, heart problems, herpes, liver problems, multiple sclerosis, Parkinson's disease, psoriasis, Raynaud's disease, seborrheic dermatitis, shingles, sinusitis,** and **vaginitis.**

A deficiency of one B vitamin usually suggests that you have low levels of others as well. People who are susceptible to a vitamin B deficiency include alcoholics, people who eat a lot of sugar, the elderly, people with malabsorption conditions or who take antibiotics for a long time, pregnant women, and nursing mothers. Signs of deficiency include scaly, oily skin, stomach distress, headache, anxiety, moodiness, and heart arrhythmias.

What to Buy: Tablets or capsules, often sold as B-50's and B-100's, which means the supplement supplies either 50 percent or 100 percent, respectively, of the DRI for each B vitamin.

How to Use: Take with food. If you are taking a multivitamin-mineral, you probably do not need a B complex unless you are treating a specific condition. See individual medical entries for specific dosages.

Possible Side Effects and Precautions: Side effects are rare and are usually seen only when the supplement is taken in extremely large amounts. Magnesium supplements can reduce absorption of B vitamins. You may need to increase your B vitamin intake when taking magnesium.

VITAMIN C Vitamin C, or ascorbic acid, is a water-soluble vitamin that is perhaps best known for its ability to help fight **colds and flu.** That's because vitamin C is a powerful antioxidant that neutralizes potentially harmful organisms and enhances the immune system. Vitamin C also helps prevent **bronchitis,** promotes wound healing, reduces the symptoms of **allergies,** prevents **cataracts,** and helps overcome **gingivitis.** On top of all that vitamin C also helps maintain tissue structure of the skin, blood vessels, bone, and gums.

A deficiency of vitamin C can cause scurvy, a disease characterized by hemorrhaging of the gums, lost teeth, anemia, joint tenderness and swelling, poor wound healing, and weakness. Scurvy is very rare in the United States. Marginally deficient levels of vitamin C, however, are sometimes seen among the elderly, hospitalized patients, and people on very restrictive diets. These individuals often are susceptible to infection and have slow wound healing.

Food sources of vitamin C include fruits and vegetables, especially citrus, tomatoes, green peppers, parsley, dark green leafy vegetables, broccoli, cantaloupe, strawberries, and potatoes. Researchers report that people absorb between 80 and 90 percent of the vitamin C they consume in their food. Factors that increase people's requirement for vitamin C include smoking, exposure to smoke or other toxic fumes, and the following conditions: burns, congestive heart disease, diarrhea, rheumatic fever, rheumatoid arthritis, trauma, surgery, and infection.

Because vitamin C is such a potent antioxidant, it is recommended for many conditions in addition to those mentioned above, including **anemia, atherosclerosis, canker sores, chronic fatigue syndrome, diabetes, ear**

infections, erectile problems, gallstones, glaucoma, hemorrhoids, herpes, high blood pressure, inflammatory bowel disease, kidney stones, macular degeneration, multiple sclerosis, osteoarthritis, psoriasis, shingles, sinusitis, ulcers, urinary-tract infections, vaginitis, and **varicose veins.**

What to Buy: Recommended forms are tablets or capsules in 500- or 1,000-mg doses for ease in dosing. Because vitamin C is eliminated from the body two to three hours after taking it, time-release formulas are preferred. Avoid the chewable tablets, because they can erode the enamel on your teeth. Also available in powder and syrup.

How to Use: Most people who take vitamin C take between 500 and 4,000 mg daily, in divided doses. Vitamin C works best along with calcium, magnesium, and bioflavonoids like quercetin. See individual medical entries for specific dosages.

Possible Side Effects and Precautions: At high doses (3,000 mg or more) some people experience diarrhea. If you or your health-care practitioner have decided you need a high dose of vitamin C, start at a low dose and increase gradually (500 to 1,000 mg increase every two days). If you experience diarrhea before you reach your target dosage, reduce your dosage the next day to the previous day's level and maintain that dosage. Vitamin C is essentially nontoxic: whatever the body can't use is excreted in the urine.

VITAMIN D Vitamin D is a unique substance in that the body produces it using sunlight on the skin. This vitamin stimulates the absorption of calcium and has anticancer properties against breast and colon cancer. A deficiency of vitamin D results in diseases that are characterized by soft, poorly formed bones—rickets in children and osteomalacia in adults. Both conditions are rare in the United States except among the elderly, who are more likely to get little or no exposure to sunlight because of ill health. The result is a loss of bone density and strength, and joint pain. The elderly population is the one group most likely to take vitamin D supplements, especially those with **osteoporosis.**

Food sources of vitamin D include cold-water fish, egg yolks, butter, and dark green leafy vegetables. Vitamin D, in the form of vitamin D_2, or ergocalciferol, is often added to milk and other foods.

What to Buy: A good-quality multivitamin-mineral usually contains an appropriate amount of vitamin D. As a single nutrient it is available in tablet and capsule. The form most often used in supplements is vitamin D_2. The prescription form of vitamin D is called calcitriol and is about ten times more potent than vitamin D_2.

How to Use: The recommended level for most people is 200 to 400 IU daily. Elderly people who do not get enough sunlight should take 400 to 800 IU daily.

Possible Side Effects and Precautions: Of all the vitamins, vitamin D has the most potential to be toxic. High intake of vitamin D (more than 1,000 IU daily) can result in kidney stones and calcium deposits in the internal organs.

VITAMIN E Vitamin E is a fat-soluble vitamin that has strong antioxidant properties. One of its primary tasks is to prevent oxidation, a chemical reaction that can cause illness, disease, and other harmful effects. Vitamin E also plays a major role in maintaining proper functioning of the muscles and nerves.

Recent studies show that vitamin E is a major factor in preventing heart problems by helping stop oxidation of cholesterol in the arteries. It appears to protect against certain **cancers,** provide relief of **fibrocystic breast disease** and **PMS,** and help maintain metabolic control in **diabe-**

tes. It is also recommended for conditions that can benefit from potent antioxidants, such as **AIDS, acne, Alzheimer's disease, atherosclerosis, backache, bronchitis, bursitis, cataracts, chronic fatigue syndrome, common cold and flu, dandruff, endometriosis, erectile problems, gallstones, hemorrhoids, high blood pressure, infertility, inflammatory bowel disease, macular degeneration, menopause, multiple sclerosis, osteoarthritis, Parkinson's disease, psoriasis, rheumatoid arthritis, seborrheic dermatitis, ulcers, vaginitis,** and **varicose veins.**

Food sources of vitamin E include various oils—sunflower, almond, wheat-germ, and hazelnut—as well as avocados, whole-grain cereals, dark green leafy vegetables, and eggs. Most people do not get a sufficient amount of vitamin E from their diet. Even so, most people do not develop symptoms of vitamin E deficiency, which include lethargy, inability to concentrate, staggering gait, loss of balance, and anemia. People most likely to experience symptoms of vitamin E deficiency are the elderly, people with chronic liver disease, or those on very low-fat diets.

What to Buy: The preferred form is natural vitamin E, which is derived from soybean or wheat-germ oil. Natural vitamin E is better absorbed than the synthetic forms, which are made from purified petroleum oil. Look for d-alpha-tocopherol on the package. Natural vitamin E comes in oil-filled capsules and dry tablets in 200- or 400-IU doses.

How to Use: Studies of vitamin E show that a level of at least 100 to 400 IU is recommended for health and prevention of disease.

Possible Side Effects and Precautions: Vitamin E does not cause any known side effects except in extremely high doses. People with rheumatic heart disease, an overactive thyroid, diabetes, or high blood pressure should consult with their physician before taking vitamin E.

YOHIMBÉ Yohimbé (*Corynanthe yohimbe*) is derived from the West African yohimbehe tree. It is used as an aphrodisiac among the Bantu tribes in Africa as well as among men in many societies, including those in the United States. It has also gained much attention as a treatment for impotence (see **erectile dysfunction**). Research has shown that yohimbé contains alkaloids, including yohimbine, which the Food and Drug Administration has recognized as the ingredient that makes yohimbé effective in the treatment of impotence.

Yohimbé works by increasing the blood flow to the penis and constricting the veins, which prevents the blood from leaving the penis and helps maintain an erection.

What to Buy: Capsules and tincture are recommended; also available as dried herb and by prescription as Yocon.

How to Use: Yohimbé should be used under supervision by a physician. For the tincture, take 15 to 20 drops in water once daily; for capsules, one 250- or 500-mg capsule daily. To make an infusion, boil 16 oz water and add 1 oz dried herb and boil for three minutes. Simmer for twenty minutes, strain the liquid, and sip slowly. To reduce the chance of nausea, add 1,000 mg vitamin C to the tea.

Possible Side Effects and Precautions: Common side effects include nausea, mild hallucinations, chills, dizziness, weakness of the limbs, nervousness, and anxiety. These effects are followed by a relaxed feeling. Yohimbé is an MAO (monoamine oxidase) inhibitor and can cause a severe decrease in blood pressure if it is taken with narcotics, antihistamines, sedatives, alcohol, tranquilizers, or dairy foods. Women should not take yohimbé. Others who should avoid it include anyone with a history of heart or kidney disease, diabetes, high or low blood pressure, duodenal or gastric ulcer, psychiatric illness, and the elderly.

ZINC   Zinc is a mineral that is critical to the work of more than three hundred enzymes in the body. These enzymes assist in cell reproduction, maintain vision, enhance the immune system, maintain fertility, repair wounds, synthesize protein, and perform many other functions. Because of its importance in so many tasks, zinc is supportive of numerous conditions, including **acne,** benign prostatic hyperplasia (see **prostate problems), common cold,** Crohn's disease (see **inflammatory bowel disease**), **diabetes, ear infections, infertility, macular degeneration, osteoporosis, rheumatoid arthritis,** and **ulcers.**

Most Americans consume less than the recommended amount of zinc, but those who are most likely to be significantly deficient are alcoholics and people with chronic kidney disease, malabsorption conditions, or sickle cell anemia.

What to Buy: Any form—tablets, lozenges, or capsules, as zinc picolinate, zinc aspartate, or zinc chelate, all of which are the most easily absorbed. Look for these forms in your multivitamin-mineral supplement as well.

How to Use: Avoid eating the following foods within two hours of taking a zinc supplement, because the body will not absorb the nutrient: bran, high-fiber foods, foods high in phosphorus such as milk and poultry, whole-grain breads and cereals. Also, if you are taking copper, iron, and/or phosphorus supplements, take them at least two hours before or after taking zinc.

Possible Side Effects and Precautions: Zinc lozenges may cause mouth irritation, nausea, stomachache, and a bad taste in some individuals. Supplementing with more than 300 mg daily may impair the immune system.

PART II

COMMON MEDICAL
CONDITIONS AND AILMENTS

This section is composed of brief, yet comprehensive, descriptions of common medical conditions, diseases, and other ailments and the most effective natural supplements you can take to help prevent, treat, or cure them. The recommended supplements listed with each condition are meant to complement conventional treatment. Conventional medicine plays a significant role in health care, and indeed, you should consult your health-care provider before beginning any type of complementary care. But the major positive impact of complementary treatments is becoming increasingly apparent to patients, physicians, and researchers. In less serious disorders (e.g., colds and flu, constipation, mild to moderate bouts of diarrhea, heartburn, or PMS), complementary remedies can often eliminate the need for conventional treatment. Many users of complementary medicine find that they can significantly reduce their dependence on conventional medications, thus reducing their risk of adverse effects. These benefits of complementary medicine are vitally important, especially given the fact that an estimated 140,000 people die each year from adverse reactions to prescription drugs that have been classified as "safe and effective" by the Food and Drug Administration, and millions suffer unnecessary negative reactions.

The suggested supplements listed with each medical condition in the pages that follow are divided into two groups: "Most Helpful Supplements" and "Other Helpful Supplements." The supplements in the "Most Helpful" category are those found to be most effective for the corresponding ailment or disease. However, everyone's body chemistry is different, which means no two people respond the exact same way to the same remedies. Please consult with your physician or another health-care practitioner who is knowledgeable about nutrition and supplementation before starting any supplement program or treatment regimen. She or he can help you decide which supplements may be best for you.

The treatment options suggested in the following pages are to be taken in addition to the recommended basic daily multivitamin-mineral supplement you choose for yourself, as described in Part III, after you allow for the amounts in the multiple. For example, say you have eczema, and you and your doctor decide to treat it with three of the four supplements classified as "Most Helpful" under the Eczema entry: licorice (2 to 4 mL fluid extract), vitamin A (5,000 IU), and zinc (45 to 60 mg). Your multivitamin-mineral contains 15 mg zinc and 5,000 IU vitamin A. Therefore, you need at least 30 mg zinc, no additional vitamin A, and a licorice supplement.

NOTE: To avoid repetition the acronym ACES is used to denote the antioxidants (see "What are antioxidants?" in Part III) vitamin A (as beta-carotene unless noted otherwise), vitamin C, vitamin E, and selenium. Their dosages are given in respective order, separated by semicolons: for example, 10,000 IU; 3,000 mg; 400 IU; 200 mg. All words in **bold** have a separate entry elsewhere in this book: supplements can be found in Part I and ailments elsewhere in Part II.

Medical Conditions and Ailments

ACNE Acne is the most common skin disorder. It usually affects the face and, to a lesser degree, the back, shoulders, and chest. Acne can appear in several different forms. *Acne vulgaris* is common among teenagers and is triggered by the surge in hormone production that occurs during adolescence. The increase in hormones in turn raises the production of sebum, a substance that lubricates the skin; and keratin, a component of hair. Excess sebum and keratin can become clogged in the hair follicles, leading to blackheads and whiteheads. Both of these skin lesions may develop into more serious types of pimples called cysts or nodules, which penetrate under the skin and may become inflamed and/or infected. This type of acne is called *acne conglobata.*

Adult-onset acne appears in people who are around thirty and older and is often caused by an allergic reaction to cosmetics or food, although some cases are related to menstruation. *Rosacea,* an acnelike condition that mostly affects women older than thirty, begins as a persistent flush on the cheeks and nose that may cause the nose to become thickened, red, and tender, especially in men.

Many people believe acne is caused by poor diet—chocolate, fried foods, and sodas—as well as inadequate hygiene and stress, yet these factors only aggravate the condition; they do not cause it. Use of contraceptives and corticosteroids, including anabolic steroids, also can contribute to, but do not cause, acne. In fact, the cause of acne is not completely understood, although it is known that heredity and hormones are involved.

Most Helpful Supplements

- **Chromium:** helps with metabolism of sugar, and impaired sugar metabolism may cause acne. Take 200 mcg chromium picolinate daily with food.
- **Pyridoxine (vitamin B$_6$):** for premenopausal acne. Take 25 to 50 mg two to three times daily.
- **Tea tree oil:** treats acne. Apply oil to affected areas once or twice daily.
- **Zinc:** relieves inflammation and heals damaged skin. Take 45 to 85 mg daily for a few months; then 30 mg daily.

Other Helpful Supplements

- **Aloe vera:** soothes the skin. Apply gel as needed daily.
- **Evening primrose oil:** helps heal damaged skin cells. Take 500 to 1,000 mg daily.
- **Lecithin:** improves absorption of the essential fatty acids, which helps repair damaged skin cells. Take 1 gel cap before each meal.
- **Vitamin E:** for overall antiacne protection. Take 400 IU daily.

AIDS Acquired immunodeficiency syndrome, or AIDS, is a disease caused by the human immunodeficiency virus, or HIV. AIDS is characterized by a severely compromised immune system. Because the immune system is weakened, individuals with AIDS are highly susceptible to countless infections and diseases. Symptoms of AIDS include long-term fatigue, prolonged fever, night sweats, unexplained weight loss, swollen lymph nodes, persistent cough or sore throat, persistent colds and diarrhea, discolored skin lesions, and bruising or bleeding that cannot be explained.

HIV is spread from person to person via infected body

fluids, such as semen, vaginal fluids, and blood, and can occur through unprotected sexual contact, during childbirth (transmitted from mother to child), through a tainted blood transfusion, or among drug users who share needles. The virus damages the body's ability to manufacture enough white blood cells, which fight infection, and thus leaves the body unable to resist invading organisms.

To date there is no cure for AIDS. The role of treatment is to slow progression of the disease, improve the quality of life, and relieve symptoms.

Most Helpful Supplements

- **Garlic:** for its antiviral and antibacterial properties. Take two 500-mg capsules three times daily with meals. ·
- **Vitamin B complex:** Take 100 mg three times daily.
- **Vitamin C:** to boost the immune system. Take 500 to 1,000 mg three times daily. Some experts recommend up to 10,000 mg as part of an ascorbic acid (vitamin C) "flush," which helps eliminate toxins in people with AIDS and other serious conditions. See sidebar for instructions.
- **Vitamin E:** antioxidant. Take 400 to 800 IU daily.

Other Helpful Supplements

- **Coenzyme Q10:** improves energy level. Take 30 to 150 mg daily.
- **Germanium:** increases oxygen to the tissues. Take 200 mg twice daily.
- **Licorice:** improves immune system function and liver function. Take any one of the following three

VITAMIN C FLUSH

Dissolve 1,000 mg (one teaspoon) ascorbic acid powder (calcium ascorbate or a similar product) in water or juice. Drink this mixture every thirty minutes until diarrhea develops. Note the amount of vitamin C you take before diarrhea occurs and subtract one teaspoon from that total. Take this new amount every four hours for up to two days. If your stools become watery, reduce the total by another teaspoon.

times daily: powdered root, 1–2 g; or fluid extract, 2–4 mL; or dry powdered extract, 250–500 mg.

- **Selenium:** destroys free radicals. Take 200 mcg daily.

ALLERGIES The word *allergy* refers to any abnormal or adverse reaction by the immune system to a substance that is generally harmless but which the body detects as foreign and threatening. Among the most common types of allergies are hay fever, asthma, food allergies, drug allergies, and insect-sting allergies, such as to bees and spiders. The body's reactions to each of these types of allergies differ, yet the primary mechanisms are the same: When the immune system perceives an offensive substance (for example, the venom from a bee sting or pollen from a flower), the body releases a chemical called histamine. The histamine triggers a series of symptoms, such as sneezing, nasal congestion, and coughing (respiratory or drug allergy); itchy throat, mouth, and eyes (respiratory allergy); stomachache, indigestion, vomiting, diarrhea (food allergy); itchy, reddening, swelling, or irritated skin (drug, food, and insect allergies); and swollen, stiff, and/or painful joints (food or drug allergy). In people with asthma another group of chemicals called leukotrienes cause asthmatic symptoms, which include swelling of the lung lining, spasm of the airway tubes, and excessive production of thick mucus. Leukotrienes are approximately one thousand times more potent than antihistamines in causing symptoms.

Most Helpful Supplements

- **Calcium:** to help reduce stress. Take 1,500 to 2,000 mg with **magnesium,** 750 mg.
- **Ephedra:** works with licorice. Take 12.5 to 25 mg two to three times daily (see **ephedra** for details) of a standardized preparation.
- **Licorice:** an antiinflammatory and antiallergic agent. Take any one of the following three times daily: 1 to 2 g powdered root; 2 to 4 mL fluid extract; 250 to 500 mg solid powdered extract.
- **Nettle:** relieves sneezing and itchy eyes. Take two to three 300-mg capsules or tablets three times daily, or 2 to 4 mL tincture three times daily.
- **Quercetin:** a bioflavonoid that is a natural antihistamine and antiasthma agent. Take 400 mg five to twenty minutes before each meal.
- **Vitamin C:** a natural antihistamine. Take 10 to 30 mg daily for every two pounds of body weight. Take in divided doses.

Other Helpful Supplements

- **Coenzyme Q10:** prevents production of histamine. Take 50 to 150 mg daily. Consult with your physician about the best dosage for you.
- **Pyridoxine (vitamin B$_6$):** effective in asthma patients. Take 25 to 50 mg twice daily.

- **Selenium:** low levels are found in asthmatics. Take 200 to 400 mg daily.
- **Vitamin B$_{12}$:** important asthma therapy. Take 1 to 3 mg daily.

ALZHEIMER'S DISEASE Alzheimer's disease is a condition in which the brain tissue deteriorates progressively, resulting in a continuous decline in mental and eventually physical abilities. The damage to the brain is characterized by two conditions: the nerve fibers in the brain become tangled, and protein deposits called plaque attach themselves to the fibers. Alzheimer's disease is more common among people age sixty-five and older, although it can affect younger individuals. The cause remains unknown, but scientists have determined that it is not a natural result of aging.

Researchers have several theories about what may cause or contribute to Alzheimer's disease. One is a blood protein called ApoE (apolipoprotein E), which has several forms. The presence of this protein is determined by genetics, and several of the forms have been associated with a higher risk of Alzheimer's. It is unclear whether ApoE destroys the nerve cells in the brain or if it is involved with plaque formation. Another theory is heredity, because individuals who have a parent with Alzheimer's are at higher risk of developing the disease. Two controversial theories are that aluminum and/or zinc cause Alzheimer's, yet these both remain unproven.

So far there is no cure for Alzheimer's disease and no known way to reverse or stop progression of the disease. A few studies suggest that estrogen may protect against it or possibly improve mental functioning, while others suggest vitamin E offers even greater protective benefit. All therapies, both conventional and natural, aim to slow the advancement of the disease and ease symptoms.

Most Helpful Supplements

- **Carnitine:** helps delay disease progression. Take 500 mg three times daily of L-acetyl-carnitine.
- **Coenzyme Q10:** helps transport oxygen to the cells and improve brain function. Take 100 mg daily.
- **Ginkgo:** alleviates anxiety, short-term memory loss, depression, inability to concentrate, and/or confusion, when taken in the early stages. Allow four to six weeks to see results. Take 40 to 80 mg three times daily.
- **Vitamin E:** helps slow disease progression. Take up to 2,000 IU daily.

Other Helpful Supplements

- **DHEA:** enhances memory, improves cognitive function. Take 25 to 50 mg for men over age fifty; 15 to 25 mg for women.
- **Lecithin:** improves brain function. Take 1 Tbs granules with meals.
- **Thiamin:** improves mental function. Take 3 to 8 grams daily.

ANEMIA Anemia is a condition in which the blood is deficient in either red blood cells or hemoglobin, which is the portion of the red blood cells that contains iron. The presence of either of these situations causes a lack of oxygen to be delivered to the tissues, and the result is fatigue, weakness, and pallor.

Anemia can be caused by excessive destruction of red blood cells, excessive loss of blood, or deficient production of red blood cells. Excessive destruction may occur when red blood cells have an abnormal shape, which is seen in sickle-cell anemia and other hereditary diseases and in vitamin and mineral deficiency. Excessive blood loss may be acute (as in a trauma situation) or chronic (e.g., a bleeding ulcer, heavy menstrual flow). Deficient red-blood-cell production is the most common category of anemia, and poor nutrition is the most common cause. The three most prevalent types of nutrient-deficient anemia are those related to a deficiency of iron, folic acid, or vitamin B_{12}. The only way to get a definite diagnosis of anemia is to get a blood test. If you suspect you have anemia, do not begin a supplement program, especially one that includes iron, until you have a diagnosis from your physician. Iron is very toxic if taken in large quantities.

Iron-deficiency anemia is seen most often in infants younger than two years old, teenage girls, pregnant women, and the elderly. Factors associated with this type of anemia include poor dietary intake of iron, reduced iron absorption or utilization, blood loss, an increased need for iron, or a combination of these situations.

Folic-acid deficiency is the most prevalent vitamin deficiency on earth. The groups most likely to have folic-acid anemia are alcoholics, pregnant women, and people with malabsorption conditions (e.g., Crohn's disease, celiac disease; see **inflammatory bowel disease**) or chronic **diarrhea.** In addition to anemia a folic-acid deficiency also causes depression, diarrhea, and a swollen, red tongue.

Most Helpful Supplements

- **Folic acid:** for folic-acid-deficiency anemia. Take 800 to 1,200 mcg folic acid three times daily plus 1,000 mcg vitamin B_{12} per day.
- **Iron:** For iron-deficiency anemia. Take 30 mg succinate, gluconate, or fumarate iron, twice a day between meals. If the iron causes stomach distress, switch to 30 mg with meals three times daily.

- **Vitamin C:** helps the body absorb iron. Take 1,000 mg three times a day with meals.
- **Vitamin B$_{12}$:** for B$_{12}$-deficiency anemia. Take 2,000 mcg sublingual three times daily for thirty days, then 1,000 mcg methylcobalamin (the active form of B$_{12}$) once per day, plus folic acid.

Other Helpful Supplements

- **Dandelion:** for iron-deficiency anemia. Take 4 to 8 mL (1 to 2 tsp) fluid extract daily.
- **Pantothenic acid (vitamin B$_5$):** helps red-blood-cell production. Take 100 mg daily.
- **Pyridoxine (vitamin B$_6$):** helps red-blood-cell production. Take 50 mg three times daily.

ATHEROSCLEROSIS/ARTERIOSCLEROSIS The phrase *hardening of the arteries* refers to two very similar conditions: arteriosclerosis, which is the accumulation of calcium deposits on the inside of artery walls; and atherosclerosis, in which the deposits are fatty substances (plaque) instead of calcium. In both cases blood circulation is restricted as it moves through hardened, narrow arteries. The restricted blood flow causes blood pressure to rise, cells to die, and eventually, often a heart attack or stroke.

Hardening of the arteries is usually associated with poor diet and lifestyle habits. Some of the main factors that contribute to arteriosclerosis and atherosclerosis are a diet that is high in fat and cholesterol and low in fiber, smoking, lack of adequate exercise, stress, being overweight, diabetes, and high blood pressure. During the early stages of arteriosclerosis and atherosclerosis, which can begin in childhood, most people notice no symptoms. Some experience a dull, cramplike pain in their legs, ankles, hip, or buttocks, which may indicate partially blocked blood vessels.

Most Helpful Supplements

- **Folic acid**: helps lower levels of homocysteine. Take 800 mcg daily, along with vitamin B_{12}.
- **Garlic**: regulates fat in the blood. Take as directed on package.
- **Hawthorn**: helps prevent plaque buildup, lowers blood pressure. Take 100 to 250 mg three times daily.
- **Inositol**: lowers cholesterol. According to Michael Murray, ND, take 1,000 to 3,000 mg daily. Supplementation should be supervised by a physician.
- **Vitamin E**: fights free radicals. Take 400 to 1,000 IU daily.
- **Vitamin C**: fights free radicals; 6,000 to 10,000 mg daily in divided doses. Also try the ascorbic acid flush. (see sidebar, p. 100).

Other Helpful Supplements

- **Fenugreek**: Take 5 to 30 g (capsules) three times a day with each meal or 15 to 90 g once daily with food; or take the tincture according to package directions.
- **Omega-3**: lowers harmful cholesterol levels. Take 1 Tbs flaxseed oil daily.
- **Quercetin**: a bioflavonoid that protects the good cholesterol (LDL) from damage and lowers the risk of heart disease. Take 35 mg daily.
- **Selenium**: promotes the benefits of vitamin E. Take 200 mcg daily.
- **Vitamin B_{12}**: helps lower levels of homocysteine. Take 100 to 300 mcg daily. Always take along with folic acid.

ATHLETE'S FOOT *Tinea pedis,* or athlete's foot, is a fungal infection that causes inflammation, itching, blisters, scaling, and burning of the feet and toes. The fungus thrives in warm, moist environments, including the inside of shoes and gym locker rooms. It is mildly contagious and can be passed along via infected skin left on towels, shower floors, and so on, but most people get athlete's foot from wearing sweaty socks and shoes. People who have taken antibiotics for two weeks or longer are susceptible to athlete's foot because the drugs kill the good bacteria that help prevent foot fungal infections.

Most Helpful Supplements

- **Garlic**: helps destroy fungus. Take two 500-mg tablets three times daily, plus place tiny slivers of fresh garlic in your shoes for several days.
- **Tea tree oil** (topical): fights fungus. Dab the oil on the affected area once daily.

Other Helpful Supplements

- **Acidophilus**: helps restore good bacteria to the body. Take one of the following forms three times daily: 1 Tbs liquid extract, 1 or 2 capsules, tablets, or softgels; or 2 Tbs powder in cool liquid.
- **Goldenseal** (topical): fights fungus. Add 6 tsp to one pint of water and soak your feet for thirty minutes twice a day.
- **Zinc**: boosts the immune system and fights fungus. Take 50 mg daily.

BACKACHE Back pain is the number-one physical complaint among men and women in the United States. The main cause of back pain is weak muscles in the back and abdomen, which is perpetuated by a sedentary lifestyle. Circumstances that contribute to weakened muscles and back pain include stress, improper lifting, poor posture, improper footwear, and sleeping on an inadequate mattress. Medical causes of backache include arthritis, curvature of the spine, a herniated disc, rheumatism, kidney and bladder problems, and bone disease.

Supplements can help relieve the pain and inflammation associated with backache and improve calcium absorption for stronger bones, but they cannot improve weak muscles. Consult with your health-care provider for exercises and movement therapies that can help improve back and abdominal muscle strength and tone.

Most Helpful Supplements

- **Boron**: improves calcium uptake. Take 3 mg daily.
- **Calcium**: improves bone strength. Take in chelated form, 1,500 to 2,000 mg. Either as a single supplement along with **magnesium,** or in a calcium/magnesium combination supplement. **Magnesium** improves bone strength. Take 700 to 1,000 mg, either as a single supplement along with calcium or in a calcium/magnesium combination supplement.
- **Vitamin B$_{12}$**: aids calcium absorption. Take 2,000 mg sublingual daily.

Other Helpful Supplements

- **Manganese**: helps heal tissue and cartilage in the back and neck. Take the gluconate form, 2 to 5 mg daily.
- **Vitamin A**: helps muscle and bone metabolism. Take 25,000 IU daily.
- **Vitamin E**: helps muscle and bone metabolism and muscle formation. Take 400 to 800 IU daily.

BRONCHITIS AND PNEUMONIA Bronchitis is inflammation, irritation, or infection of the breathing tubes, or bronchi, in the upper part of the lungs. Pneumonia is an infection or irritation of the lungs. Both conditions usually follow a bout of common cold, flu, or other respiratory insult.

Bronchitis comes in two forms. Acute bronchitis has a viral cause in 90 percent of cases and is characterized by a hacking cough, fever, chills, tightness in the chest, and a yellow, green, or white phlegm that usually appears twenty-four to forty-eight hours after the cough begins. Chronic bronchitis is more serious and usually develops in people who are overweight, sedentary, and exposed to smoke. Symptoms include a persistent cough that results in yellow, green, or white phlegm that lasts for at least three months of the year and for more than two consecutive years. People with chronic bronchitis are at high risk of developing heart disease and more serious lung disease.

Pneumonia can be caused by bacteria, fungi, or viruses, and usually develops in people who have a weakened immune system, such as hospitalized patients or elderly individuals with chronic medical conditions. Symptoms of pneumonia include fever, chills, cough, muscle aches, swollen lymph glands, fatigue, sore throat, chest pains, and difficulty breathing.

Most Helpful Supplements

- **Beta-carotene**: protects the lungs. Take 15,000 to 200,000 IU daily.
- **Quercetin**: a bioflavonoid. Take 1,000 mg daily in divided doses, along with vitamin C.
- **Vitamin C**: antioxidant. Take 3,000 to 10,000 mg daily in divided doses (every two hours).
- **Zinc**: helps bronchial healing. Take 50 mg daily. Some experts recommend taking one lozenge (23 mg) every two waking hours for one week.

Other Helpful Supplements

- **Echinacea**: enhances the immune system. Take any one of the following forms three times daily: 0.5 to 1 g dried root (as a decoction); 2 to 4 mL tincture; 2 to 4 mL fluid extract; 150 to 300 mg dry powdered extract.
- **Ephedra**: opens up the bronchi. Use it in combination with other herbs—5 g ephedra, 4 g cinnamon sticks, and 1.5 g licorice. Steep the herbs in cold water, then bring to a boil. Take it hot.
- **Garlic**: natural antibiotic. Take 2 tablets with meals.
- **Vitamin E**: heals tissues and improves breathing. Take 400 IU twice daily.

BURSITIS AND TENDINITIS Inflammation of the bursae, fluid-filled sacs that cushion the bones, ligaments, and tendons when they move against each other, is known as bursitis. Inflammation in or around a tendon is tendinitis. Both of these conditions involve pain, inflammation, and swelling and can restrict movement, but they do differ somewhat. Bursitis commonly affects the shoulders, elbows, hips, knees, and the joints in the feet and hands. The symptoms are especially apparent when lifting, stretching, or whenever a joint is moved repetitively or beyond its normal range of motion.

In tendinitis the tendons become inflamed when they are overused, either repetitively or occasionally. The areas most often affected are the shoulder, wrist, heel, and elbow (tennis elbow). Other symptoms include stiffness and, in some cases, swelling, tingling, or numbness.

Most Helpful Supplements

- **Boswellia**: for inflammation. Take 150 mg three times daily.

- **Bromelain**: antiinflammatory. Take 250 to 750 mg three times daily between meals.
- **Vitamin C**: helps produce collagen, which builds tissue. Take 1,000 mg daily.

Other Helpful Supplements

- **Sulfur (MSM)**: relieves inflammation and pain. Take 500 to 5,000 mg daily. Start with a low dosage and increase by 500 mg every few days until you notice results.
- **Vitamin E**: heals tissues. Take 400 IU daily.
- **Zinc**: helps produce collagen, which builds tissue. Take 22.5 mg for tendinitis.

CANCER Cancer is the uncontrolled reproduction of cells that results in an abnormality, most often a tumor or similar growth. The basic cause of any of the more than one hundred different diseases classified as cancer is a mutation, or change, in the nucleus of a cell. Although the exact reasons why cells undergo this mutation process are not known, researchers have identified many substances, called carcinogens, that either start or stimulate the process. A few of the items included in this group are cigarette smoke, radiation, sunlight, excess alcohol, and chemicals in pesticides, paints, food, water, and cleaning products. Diet has been identified as a major cause of and contributor to cancer.

Cancer falls into four main categories: carcinomas, which affect the glands, skin, mucous membranes, and other organs; leukemias, which are cancers of the blood; lymphomas, which attack the lymphatic system; and sarcomas, which appear in the bones, connective tissue, and muscles.

Because there is no known cure, the following supplement treatment options target prevention of cancer, especially for people who are at risk for particular types of cancer because of family or personal history or lifestyle (e.g., smoking, alcohol abuse).

Most Helpful Supplements

- **ACES**: (as beta–carotene) 10,000 IU beta–carotene/ 5,000–10,000 mg vitamin C/1,000 IU vitamin E/ 200 mcg selenium.
- **Astragalus**: boosts the immune system and is useful following chemotherapy. To enhance the immune system, take the dried root capsules with meals or water—250 to 500 mg two to three times daily, or 3 to 5 mL ($^{1}/_{8}$ to $^{1}/_{2}$ tsp) tincture or extract three times daily. Following chemotherapy, take two to three 500-mg capsules three times daily.

Other Helpful Supplements

- **Coenzyme Q10**: promotes oxygenation of cells. Take 100 mg daily.
- **Garlic**: enhances the immune system. Take 2 capsules three times daily.
- **Green tea**: boosts the immune system. Drink up to 5 cups tea daily, preferably with meals, or take 500-mg capsules daily.

CANKER SORES Canker sores (*aphthous stomatitis*) are small, painful ulcers that develop on the inside of the mouth, alone or in small clusters. As many as 50 percent of Americans get canker sores each year. Women are twice as likely to develop them, especially before their menstrual period begins. Most canker sores go away after a few days, but they recur in many people.

The cause of canker sores is unknown, although experts believe stress plays a role, as well as a deficiency of iron, vitamin B_{12}, vitamin B_1 (thiamin), and/or folic acid. Other possible causes include a weakened immune system and food allergy. Food sensitivities can irritate canker sores.

Most Helpful Supplements

- **Licorice**: promotes healing. Take 200 mg powdered deglycyrrhizinated licorice dissolved in 200 mL warm water. Swish in the mouth for two minutes three to four times daily. Or chew a 380-mg chewable tablet twenty minutes before meals.
- **Myrrh**: promotes healing. Take 200 to 300 mg extract or 4 mL tincture with 2 to 3 oz warm water. Swish in the mouth for several minutes and swallow. Repeat two to three times daily.
- **Vitamin B complex**: promotes healing and maintains B vitamin balance. Take 50 mg three times daily.

Other Helpful Supplements

- **Acidophilus**: reduces soreness. Chew four tablets three times daily until the sores heal.
- **Dandelion**: prevents recurrence and heals sores. Take 500- to 1,000-mg capsules three times daily for six weeks.
- **Echinacea**: promotes healing. Take 4 mL liquid extract echinacea swished in the mouth for two to three minutes three times daily. Swallow the extract for added protection.
- **Vitamin C**: antioxidant. Take 3,000 to 8,000 mg daily in divided doses.

CARPAL TUNNEL SYNDROME Carpal tunnel syndrome is an increasingly common disorder that is marked by pain, weakness, numbness, tingling, and burning in the wrist and fingers that often radiates to the forearm and shoulder. It is caused by compression of the median nerve, which controls the movement of the fingers and thumb. The median nerve runs from the forearm to the fingertips and lies between the ligaments and bones of the wrist. People who perform a lot of repetitive movement of the hand, such as typists, assembly-line workers, keyboard operators, cashiers, and carpenters, are among those most likely to suffer with this condition.

Preventive measures include wearing a specially made splint for the hand and wrist, using a wrist pad when typing or keyboarding, and taking frequent breaks to exercise the wrist and hand. Studies into the use of vitamin B_6 as treatment for carpal tunnel syndrome have resulted in mixed findings. Generally, vitamin B_6 helps some patients, especially when it is combined with supplements of vitamin B_2 and other B vitamins. In any case, treatment with vitamin B_6 is safe and recommended before opting for surgery.

Most Helpful Supplements

- **Bromelain**: relieves pain and inflammation. Take 250 to 750 mg twice daily (1,200 to 1,800 mcu/gdu) between meals.
- **Pyridoxine (vitamin B_6)**: Take 25 mg three to four times daily.
- **Vitamin B complex**: enhances effectiveness of vitamin B_6. Take 50 mg once daily.

CATARACTS Cataracts are cloudy white blemishes in the lens of the eye that obstruct vision. They affect approximately 4 million Americans and are the number-one cause of vision impairment and blindness in the United States.

Cataracts form because of damage to the protein structure of the lens by free radicals. Therefore intake of antioxidants is one way to prevent and treat cataracts. In particular, vitamin C can stop cataract formation and even improve vision in some individuals. The antioxidants vitamin E and selenium, as well as the herb **bilberry,** also have proven effective in preventing and treating cataracts.

Senile cataracts, which affect persons sixty-five years and older, are the most common form of this eye disease. Free-radical damage to the lens is the main cause of this form of cataracts. Other conditions and situations that contribute to the formation of cataracts include diabetes, exposure to radiation or toxins, eye trauma, eye diseases, eye surgery, and hereditary factors. To help prevent cataracts and avoid further damage when cataracts are already present, people should wear sunglasses that provide ultraviolet-light protection when outdoors.

Most Helpful Supplements

- **ACES**: 200,000 IU daily; 1,000 mg vitamin C three times daily; 400 to 800 IU vitamin E, take with bilberry; 400 mcg selenium daily.
- **Bilberry**: protection against cataract formation and progression. Take 40 to 80 mg extract three times daily; take with vitamin E.

Other Helpful Supplements

- **Copper**: promotes healing and retards growth of cataracts. Take 3 mg daily; take with zinc.
- **Quercetin**: bioflavonoid. Take 500 mg three times daily.
- **Selenium**: low levels promote cataract formation. Take 400 mcg daily; take with vitamin E.
- **Vitamin B complex**: promotes overall cell health. Take 50 mg daily.
- **Vitamin B$_2$ (riboflavin)**: deficiency linked to cataract formation. Take 50 mg daily.
- **Zinc**: promotes healing and retards growth of cataracts. Take 50 mg daily; take with copper.

CHRONIC FATIGUE SYNDROME Chronic fatigue syndrome (CFS) is a term that describes a group of symptoms, including persistent and recurrent fatigue, low-grade fever, swollen lymph nodes, muscle weakness, headache, muscle and joint pain, sore throat, depression, and loss of concentration. Symptoms of chronic fatigue syndrome are similar to those of other conditions, especially **fibromyalgia** and multiple chemical sensitivity disorder.

Chronic fatigue syndrome was formally defined by the Centers for Disease Control in 1988, and diagnostic criteria were established. Despite this more recent recognition of the condition, chronic fatigue syndrome apparently was identified first in the 1860s and has since then been called various names, including chronic mononucleosislike syndrome, Yuppie flu, and postinfectious neuromyasthenia.

The cause of chronic fatigue syndrome is uncertain. One possibility is the Epstein–Barr virus (EBV), which is a member of a larger group of herpesviruses. EBV is suspect because, similar to other viruses in the herpes group, it remains dormant in the body until the immune system becomes weakened. At that time the virus can become active and cause symptoms typical of CFS. Other organisms also have been named as possible causes of CFS, including herpesvirus-6, brucella, and enterovirus.

There are many ways the immune system can become impaired: stress, poor diet, insufficient sleep, smoking, alcohol or drug use. A deficiency of nearly any nutrient can make the immune system susceptible to invasion by harmful organisms that can greatly weaken the body and cause fatigue.

Chronic fatigue alone can have many causes and not necessarily be associated with CFS. Some of the major causes of chronic fatigue include the presence of yeast infection, diabetes, heart disease, rheumatoid arthritis, lung disease, chronic pain, cancer, liver disease, and multiple sclerosis. Depression, high levels of stress, food allergies, anemia, as well as use of antihypertensive drugs, tranquilizers, birth control pills, antiinflammatory medications, and antihistamines are also linked with chronic fatigue.

Most Helpful Supplements

- **Astragalus**: strengthens the immune system. Take 250 to 500 mg dried root capsules two to three times daily with meals or water, or 3 to 5 mL ($^1/_8$ to $^1/_2$ tsp) tincture or extract three times daily.
- **Coenzyme Q10**: boosts the immune system. Take 75 mg daily.
- **Ginseng (Siberian)**: strengthens the immune system. Take any of the following three times daily: dried root, 2 to 4 g; 10 to 20 mL tincture; 2 to 4 mL fluid extract; 100 to 200 mg dry powdered extract.
- **Licorice**: antiviral. Take any one of the following three times daily: 2 to 4 g powdered root; 2 to 4 mL fluid extract; 250 to 500 mg dry powdered extract. People with chronic fatigue syndrome who have adrenal insufficiency or abnormally low blood pressure are most likely to benefit from licorice.
- **Vitamin C**: antiviral. Take 1,000 to 3,000 mg three times daily.
- **Vitamin E**: antioxidant. Take 400 to 800 IU daily for one month, then gradually decrease to 400 IU daily. An emulsion is preferred over pills.

Other Helpful Supplements

- **Acidophilus**: restores "good" bacteria in those with candida infection. Take 1 to 2 billion CFU daily.
- **Lecithin**: boosts the immune system and promotes energy. Take 1 Tbs granules that are 20 percent phosphatidylcholine three times daily with food.

- **Magnesium**: relieves fatigue and muscle pain. Take magnesium citrate or aspartate, 200 to 300 mg three times daily.

COLDS AND FLU The common cold and influenza, or flu, can be caused by a wide variety of viruses that attack the upper respiratory system. Although cold and flu affect nearly all people at least once in their lifetime, they are hard to cure because the viruses easily and quickly change size and shape. This has made it impossible thus far to develop vaccines that completely eliminate colds and flu.

Symptoms of common cold include general malaise, headache, upper-respiratory-tract congestion, sneezing, watery eyes, nasal discharge, sore throat, and fever. Symptoms of flu are similar to those of the common cold and usually also include muscular aches and pain, chills, and fatigue. Nausea and vomiting may also occur.

Most of the symptoms of cold and flu are the body's attempt to rid itself of the infectious organisms. Therefore, taking a nasal decongestant to eliminate nasal discharge, for example, is not helpful because it prevents the body from ridding itself of the virus. Natural remedies for cold and flu are geared to boost the immune system and help the body shed the virus, which ultimately results in symptom relief. Along with the treatment options mentioned below, rest and consumption of large amounts of fluids (herbal tea, water, broth, and diluted juices) are recommended to help eliminate the virus.

Most Helpful Supplements

- **Astragalus**: boosts the immune system. Take 250 to 500 mg dried root capsules two to three times daily with food or water, or 3 to 5 mL ($1/8$ to $1/2$ tsp) extract or tincture three times daily.
- **Echinacea**: enhances the immune system. Take any

one of the following forms three times daily: 0.5 to 1 g dried root (as a tea); 2 to 4 mL tincture; 2 to 4 mL fluid extract; 150 to 300 mg dry powdered extract.

- **Vitamin A**: heals inflamed membranes and boosts immune system. Take 15,000 to 25,000 IU for up to four days.
- **Vitamin C**: helps destroy the virus. Take 500 to 1,000 mg every two hours (as tolerated) daily.
- **Zinc**: antiviral, also relieves sore throat. Dissolve 1 lozenge (15 to 25 mg each) of elemental zinc under the tongue every three hours the first three days, then one every four hours for up to another four days. Do not take zinc for longer than seven days. For flu, dissolve 1 lozenge every two hours for up to one week.

Other Helpful Supplements

- **Beta-carotene**: boosts the immune system. Take 50,000 to 100,000 IU daily.
- **Garlic**: enhances the immune system. Take 2 capsules 3 times daily.
- **Myrrh**: effective antibacterial. Take 1 capsule three times daily or 1 to 2 mL tincture three times daily.
- **Quercetin**: destroys the virus. Take 1,000 mg with each dose of vitamin C.

CONSTIPATION Constipation occurs when solid waste material, or stool, moves too slowly through the intestinal tract. The result is hard, compacted stools that are painful when passed. Other symptoms that may accompany constipation include gas, stomach pain, headache, indigestion, and bad breath.

Normal stool is neither too hard nor too soft and is eliminated every eighteen to twenty-four hours. People with constipation may have a bowel movement once every two to three days and strain to pass dry stools. Frequent bouts of constipation may lead to other problems, such as hemorrhoids and varicose veins.

Constipation is usually the result of an insufficient intake of fiber and/or fluids, although occasionally it is caused by certain drugs or supplements such as iron tablets, antidepressants, and some painkillers. Constipation is also common during pregnancy. Chronic constipation may indicate a more serious condition, such as irritable bowel syndrome, colorectal cancer, multiple sclerosis, diabetes, or Parkinson's disease. If you suffer with chronic constipation, see your physician.

Occasional episodes of constipation can be treated by increasing intake of fluids and fiber, getting more exercise, and, if needed, taking a natural laxative, many of which are made from plants. Herbal laxatives work in one of two ways: they either stimulate the bowel muscles to contract, or they promote the formation of stool. Stimulant laxatives are better for acute cases of constipation, while bulk-forming laxatives are best for long-term treatment, which is often needed for people in nursing homes or bedridden patients.

Most Helpful Supplements

- **Aloe vera**: a potent stimulant laxative that helps form soft stools and promotes healing. Drink ½ cup aloe vera juice in the morning and evening, or take a 50- to 200-mg latex tablet or softgel once a day up to ten days as needed.
- **Fenugreek**: bulk-forming laxative. Take 5 to 30 g with each meal, or 30 to 90 g once daily; capsules are easier to take because the seeds are bitter.
- **Psyllium**: bulk-forming laxative. Take 7.5 g of seeds or 5 g husks, mixed with water or juice, 1 to 2 times daily.

Other Helpful Supplements

- **Dandelion**: stimulant. Take 500 to 1,000 mg fluid extract daily.
- **Sulfur (MSM)**: eliminates toxins in the colon. Take 2,000 mg daily in divided doses.

DANDRUFF Dandruff is characterized by flaking and scaling of dead skin from the scalp. This condition may be itchy and occasionally is accompanied by a scaly rash, **seborrheic dermatitis.**

When the proteins and fats in the scalp function properly, they maintain circulation of water and oils and keep the skin and hair healthy. Dandruff develops when the sebaceous glands in the scalp cannot adequately assimilate proteins and fats. Occasionally dandruff is caused by an imbalance in the kidneys or liver, two organs that are responsible for eliminating toxins from the body.

Diet plays a significant role in the control of dandruff. Recommendations include elimination of meat, dairy products, eggs, seafood, fried foods, nuts, citrus, sugar, excess salt, and alcohol.

Most Helpful Supplements

- **Tea tree oil**: prevents flaking and infection. Massage a few drops into the scalp daily.
- **Vitamin B complex**: helps break down fatty acids. Take 100 mg twice daily with meals.
- **Vitamin E**: improves circulation. Take 400 IU daily.

Other Helpful Supplements

- **Evening primrose oil**: relieves inflammation. Take two 500-mg capsules three times daily.
- **Zinc**: promotes protein metabolism (scalp is mainly

protein). Take 5 tablets dissolved in mouth daily for one week.

DEPRESSION Depression is a state of feeling hopeless and sad in response to situations that can fall into two main categories: endogenous, which refers to internal problems such as a hormone imbalance, food allergy, nutritional deficiency, or chemical abnormality as the cause of the depression; or exogenous, which means events outside oneself trigger the depression. Nutritional supplements are more effective in treating endogenous rather than exogenous depression.

Food has a significant impact on how the brain operates, particularly on the neurotransmitters, which are responsible for behavior. Production of the neurotransmitter serotonin, for example, promotes calm, and foods rich in complex carbohydrates aid functioning of serotonin. Increased levels of dopamine and norepinephrine enhance alertness, and these neurotransmitters are prompted by consumption of protein foods.

Symptoms of depression include loss of interest in everyday events, people, and things that normally give people pleasure; insomnia or a desire to sleep all the time; headache; chronic fatigue syndrome; intestinal disorders; loss of appetite or a ravenous appetite; feelings of hopelessness, inadequacy, and helplessness; and sometimes thoughts of death and suicide. Many women who have PMS experience depression as part of the syndrome.

Most Helpful Supplements

- **St. John's wort**: for mild to moderate depression. Take 250 to 300 mg two to three times daily of standardized form 0.3% hypericin.
- **Folic acid**: deficiency can disturb mood. Take 400 mcg daily.

- **5-HTP**: helps raise serotonin levels. Take 100 to 200 mg three times daily.
- **Inositol**: improves circulation in the brain. Take 100 mg twice daily along with niacin and niacinamide.
- **Niacin**: improves circulation in the brain. Take 100 mg three times daily, along with niacinamide and inositol.
- **Niacinamide (vitamin B$_3$)**: improves circulation in the brain. Take 200 mg daily, plus niacin and inositol.
- **Pyridoxine (vitamin B$_6$)**: take if deficient. Take 50 mg three times daily.
- **Vitamin B$_{12}$**: deficiency creates mood disturbances; 1,000 mcg daily after deficiency has been corrected by injections, administered by a health-care practitioner.

DIABETES Diabetes mellitus is a disease characterized by the inability to properly process and utilize sugar, or glucose, which the body uses for energy. This problem occurs because the pancreas is unable to produce a sufficient amount of the hormone insulin, which the cells need to take in and use glucose.

The two major types of diabetes are type I, or insulin-dependent diabetes, and type II, or noninsulin-dependent diabetes. People with type I diabetes do not produce insulin and so must take daily doses of insulin to help glucose enter the body's cells and tissues and provide energy. Type I diabetes nearly always first appears in childhood. Symptoms include abnormal thirst, nausea or vomiting, weakness, frequent need to urinate, irritability, fatigue, and increased appetite.

Individuals with Type II diabetes do produce insulin, but it may be an insufficient amount or the body is unable to process it effectively. Type II diabetes first occurs in adulthood and in most cases can be controlled by consuming a nutritious diet, maintaining a healthy weight, and following a routine exericise program. The majority of people with Type II diabetes, however, are obese and many take antidiabetic medication daily.

NOTE: Diabetes is a condition for which there are a multitude of natural remedies that have proved effective. Thus the number of options listed here is greater than for most of the other conditions in this section. It is important to work with a medical professional when taking any of these supplements, as their use may significantly decrease or eliminate your need for antidiabetic medications.

Most Helpful Supplements

- **Chromium**: improves glucose tolerance. Take 200 to 1,000 mcg daily.
- **Fenugreek**: regulates insulin. Researchers have used 15 to 100 g fenugreek powder daily to treat people with noninsulin-dependent diabetes. Do not take fenugreek without the guidance of a medical professional.
- **Inositol**: helps maintain normal nerve function. Take 500 mg twice daily.
- **Magnesium**: improves insulin production. Take 300 to 400 mg daily.
- **Manganese**: diabetics have half the manganese levels of normal individuals. Take 30 mg daily.

Other Helpful Supplements

- **Biotin**: promotes processing of glucose. Take 9 to 16 mg daily, under a doctor's supervision.
- **Brewer's yeast**: contains chromium. Take 1/2 to 2 Tbs two to three times daily or 1 tablet three times daily.
- **L-Carnitine**: diabetes may be associated with a defi-

ciency. Take 2 to 4 capsules or tablets daily thirty minutes before or after meals.

- **Coenzyme Q10**: aids carbohydrate metabolism. Take 120 mg daily.
- **Pyridoxine (vitamin B$_6$)**: improves glucose tolerance. Take a special form of B$_6$, called pyridoxine alpha-ketoglutarate, 1,800 mg daily.
- **Vitamin C**: protects the eyes, kidneys, and nerves. Take 1,000 to 3,000 mg daily.
- **Vitamin E**: improves glucose tolerance. Take 900 IU daily.

DIARRHEA Diarrhea is the presence of frequent watery or very loose stools. It is often a temporary condition that resolves itself within two to four days, but occasionally it is an indication of a more serious problem.

Diarrhea is not a disease but a symptom of an underlying problem, which may be caused by dietary or nondietary factors. One common trigger of diarrhea is dairy products, caused by an intolerance for the milk sugar called lactose. A deficiency of folic acid or zinc has been linked with bouts of diarrhea, as has excessive (more than 2,000 or 3,000 mg) amounts of vitamin C. Consumption of foods that contain the natural sweetener called sorbitol is also known to cause diarrhea. Nondietary causes include use of certain drugs, such as antibiotics (especially tetracycline), antacids that contain magnesium salts, or laxatives that contain magnesium, phosphate, or sulfate. People with medical conditions such as Crohn's disease, ulcerative colitis, hepatitis, or cancer typically experience diarrhea, while infection by bacteria, viruses, or parasites also causes watery stools.

Because diarrhea causes the body to lose a great deal of water and essential nutrients, individuals should replace them by drinking lots of herbal tea, fruit and vegetable juices, vegetable broth, or electrolyte-replacement drinks, which supply chloride, potassium, and sodium. Milk and dairy products should be avoided.

The most helpful remedy depends on the cause of the diarrhea. If you don't know the cause, the first two supplements should be beneficial.

Most Helpful Supplements

- **Acidophilus**: replaces "good" bacteria and is a good general remedy. Take 1 tsp powder in distilled water twice daily.
- **Brewer's yeast**: relieves infectious diarrhea. Take 3 capsules or tablets three times daily for two weeks.
- **Folic acid**: reduces recovery time and heals the intestinal walls. Take 5,000 mcg three times daily for two to three days.

Other Helpful Supplements

- **Garlic**: kills parasites and bacteria. Take 2 capsules three times daily.
- **Goldenseal**: for diarrhea caused by parasites. Take 4 to 6 g powdered root capsules daily or 4 to 6 mL liquid extract daily.
- **Potassium**: replaces potassium lost. Take 99 mg daily.

DIVERTICULITIS Diverticulitis is a disease of the colon (large intestine) in which sacs develop in the walls of the intestine and extend out into the surrounding body cavities. When particles become lodged in the sacs, the colon becomes inflamed and infection can move in. Symptoms of diverticulitis include fever, severe pain in the lower abdomen, nausea, diarrhea, and/or constipation. Some patients have no symptoms at all for years before having an attack with pain. In severe cases the disease progresses to a potentially fatal stage called peritonitis.

Individuals at high risk of developing diverticulitis include those who are obese or who have a poor diet (low fiber, high fat), family history of the disease, gallbladder disease, or coronary artery disease. It is estimated that 50 percent or more of Americans age fifty or older have diverticulitis. Supplements can be effective in mild to moderate cases of diverticulitis and can serve as complementary treatment for people with more serious cases.

Most Helpful Supplements

- **Acidophilus**: restores "good" bacteria. Take 1 tsp three times daily on an empty stomach.
- **Aloe vera**: helps to gently clean the intestinal tract. Take 1 tsp gel after meals. Don't take more, because it can act as a laxative.
- **Psyllium**: supplies fiber, which softens the stools and cleans the intestines. Take 1 tsp in water once or twice daily.

Other Helpful Supplements

- **Garlic**: promotes healing. Take 2 capsules with meals.
- **Vitamin B complex**: promotes healing. Take 100 mg three times daily.

EAR INFECTIONS Ear infections are painful conditions of the inner or outer ear, which tend to recur and typically affect children more than adults. In fact, approximately 95 percent of children experience ear infections by the time they reach age six.

One of the main types of ear infection is otitis media, or infection of the middle ear, which is very common among infants and children. Symptoms include pain in the middle ear, fever that may reach 103 degrees or higher, and a feeling of pressure in the ear. A severe middle-ear infection can lead to a ruptured eardrum. Another common type is otitis externa, or outer-ear infection, in which the area from the eardrum to the outside of the ear becomes inflamed. This type is also known as swimmer's ear. Symptoms include fever, temporary loss of hearing in the affected ear, and a discharge from the ear.

Researchers have found a definite link between food allergies and recurrent ear infection, especially chronic otitis media. More than half of children with recurrent ear infections have food allergies. When the culprit foods (milk, wheat, and eggs are the most common allergens) are eliminated, more than 75 percent of children improve significantly. Other factors associated with ear infection include exposure to secondhand smoke, smoke from wood-burning stoves, and being bottle-fed or having been breast-fed for less than four months.

Most Helpful Supplements

(Note: These dosages are for adults; consult your physician for children's doses.)

- **Echinacea:** reduces risk of infection. Take 40 drops tincture two to three times daily for six to eight weeks.
- **Vitamin A:** promotes healing. Take 50,000 IU as emulsion.
- **Vitamin C:** boosts immune response. Take 3,000 to 7,000 mg daily in divided doses.
- **Zinc:** boosts immune response. Take 10 mg as a lozenge three times daily for five days.

Other Helpful Supplements

- **Manganese:** eliminates the deficiency associated with ear infection. Take 10 mg daily.
- **Pyridoxine (vitamin B₆):** promotes healing and relieves pressure. Take 50 mg daily.

ECZEMA Approximately 2 to 7 percent of Americans have eczema (atopic dermatitis), a chronic skin condition characterized by itchy, inflamed, dry skin. Eczema is at least partially caused by allergies, proven by the fact that all people with eczema test positive on allergy tests and most improve when they consume a diet that eliminates common food allergens such as eggs, wheat, milk, and peanuts. Other characteristics shared by most people with eczema are dry, thickened skin that has very limited capacity to hold water; an overgrowth of bacteria, especially *Staphylococcus aureus,* which is found in 90 percent of patients; and a tendency for the skin to thicken when rubbed or scratched.

Nutritional and supplemental treatment of eczema focuses on preventing the release of excess histamine that is associated with allergic reactions and providing nutrients that offer antiinflammatory and antiallergic benefits. Deficiencies often seen in people with eczema include zinc and gamma-linolenic acid (GLA), a fatty acid. People with eczema do not have the ability to properly process fatty acids.

Most Helpful Supplements

- **Evening primrose oil:** restores GLA levels. Take two 500-mg capsules three times daily.
- **Licorice:** antiinflammatory and antiallergy. Take one of the following three times daily: 1 to 2 g powdered root, 2 to 4 mL fluid extract, or 250 to 500 mg dry powdered extract.

- **Vitamin A:** helps repair damaged skin. Take 5,000 IU daily.
- **Zinc:** restores low zinc levels usually seen in patients with eczema and promotes tissue repair. Take 45 to 60 mg daily, reduced to 30 mg when eczema clears.

Other Helpful Supplements

- **Dandelion:** relieves itching. Take one of the following three times a day: an infusion, prepared by simmering 1 Tbs dried root in 8 oz boiling water for ten minutes, strain and drink; take 4 to 8 mL fluid extract; or take 250 to 500 mg powdered solid extract.
- **Green tea:** antihistamine and antiallergy. Take 200 to 300 mg three times daily, or take quercetin.
- **Oats:** soothes the itch. Place 1 to 3 cups raw oats into a muslin bag and place the bag into your hot bathwater. Soak in the bathwater for fifteen to twenty minutes. An alternative method is to boil 1 pound shredded oat straw in 2 quarts of water for thirty minutes and then add the strained liquid to your bathwater.
- **Quercetin:** a bioflavonoid that is an antihistamine and antiallergy agent. Take 400 mg twenty minutes before meals; or take green tea.
- **Vitamin E:** antioxidant. Take 400 IU daily.

ENDOMETRIOSIS Approximately 10 percent of women experience endometriosis, a condition in which the cells that grow in the lining of the uterus, or the endometrium, also grow on the outside of the uterus. These cells attach and form abnormal tissue in or on the fallopian tubes, bladder, ovaries, bowel, and on the pelvic floor. Symptoms of endometriosis include severe pain in the uterus, lower back, and within the pelvic area before and during menses; painful intercourse; passing of blood clots and heavy blood flow during menses; and constipation, nausea, and vomiting during menses. Some women with endometriosis are infertile, and many have iron-deficient **anemia** because of the excessive loss of blood.

Researchers have not definitively identified the cause of endometriosis. Some believe excess endometrial cells travel through the blood and lymph channels and attach outside the uterus; others propose that some menstrual blood may back up into the fallopian tubes and leak into the area outside the uterus. Risk factors for endometriosis include never having been pregnant, use of an IUD, a consistently short menstrual cycle (less than twenty-five days), heavy menstrual flow, tampon use, and a menstrual flow that lasts more than one week.

Most Helpful Supplements

(Note: These supplements may provide relief if the condition is diagnosed and treated early.)

- **Dong quai:** regulates hormones. Take 500 mg daily in tablets or capsules.
- **Evening primrose oil:** fatty acids and GLA. Take two 500-mg capsules three times daily.
- **Pantothenic acid (vitamin B_5):** builds red blood cells; 100 mg three times daily.
- **Pyridoxine (vitamin B_6):** helps balance water levels. Take 50 mg three times daily.
- **Vitamin B complex:** promotes production of blood cells and balances hormones. Take 1 capsule daily.

Other Helpful Supplements

- **Black cohosh:** try if dong quai or chaste berry is not effective. Helps balance hormones. Take $1/2$ tsp powdered root boiled in 8 oz water for thirty minutes, then take 2 tsp at a time throughout the day until entirely consumed.

- **Chaste berry:** try if dong quai or black cohosh is not effective. Helps balance hormones. Take 2 to 3 g daily as capsules or tablets.
- **Iron:** to replace iron lost in heavy menstruation. Do not take iron supplements unless you are under a doctor's care.
- **Vitamin E:** helps balance hormone levels. Take 400 IU daily, slowly increased to 1,000 IU.

ERECTILE DYSFUNCTION (IMPOTENCE) Men who have an inability to attain and maintain an erection that is sufficient to allow penetration and satisfactory sexual intercourse have what is more correctly called erectile dysfunction, and commonly called impotence. An estimated 10 to 20 million American men experience this problem, and the number is growing as the population of baby boomers reaches midlife.

Approximately 85 percent of cases of impotence have an organic cause. For nearly 50 percent of men over the age of fifty who have erectile dysfunction, **atherosclerosis** of the penile artery is the main cause. Some of the other common causes include low levels of male sex hormones, **diabetes,** use of some medications (e.g., antihistamines, antidepressants, tranquilizers, antihypertensives), alcohol consumption, smoking, hypothyroidism, peripheral vascular disease, and prostate disorders.

Natural steps to help treat impotence include eating foods high in zinc (e.g., pumpkin seeds, nuts) and avoiding animal fats, fried foods, and sugar. Excessive exercise can contribute to impotency, but moderate exercise can help by improving circulation.

Most Helpful Supplements

- **Vitamin C:** promotes health of sperm. Take 3,000 to 6,000 mg daily in divided doses.
- **Vitamin E:** for hormone production. Take 400 to 1,000 IU daily. Start with 200 IU and increase gradually.
- **Zinc:** for prostate gland health. Take 80 mg daily.

Other Helpful Supplements

- **DHEA:** promotes vitality. Take 25 to 50 mg daily (see DHEA in Part I).
- **Ginkgo biloba:** improves penile blood flow. Take 40 mg three times daily of standardized 24 percent ginkgo flavoglycosides.
- **Ginseng:** increases sperm production and testosterone levels. Take Asian ginseng, 100 mg of root powder or extract with 5 percent ginsenosides, one to three times daily.

FIBROCYSTIC BREAST DISEASE Up to 50 percent of women have fibrocystic breast disease, a term that covers several benign (noncancerous) conditions that affect the breast. Women with fibrocystic breast disease experience tenderness or pain as well as lumps in both breasts. The lumps, or cysts, move freely in the breast, are either firm or soft, and may change in size. Pain results as the cysts fill with fluid and the tissue around them becomes thick, placing pressure on the surrounding area. This fluid is normally reabsorbed by the breast tissue, but as a woman ages the ability of the lymph system to absorb the fluid decreases, and cysts remain. The cysts are most painful before menstruation.

Fibrocystic breast disease appears to be caused by an imbalance in the ratio of estrogen to progesterone, as well as changes in the levels of other hormones. Consumption of caffeine, theobromine, and theophylline are also known to cause the formation of fibrous tissue and the production of cyst fluid in the breast. These three compounds, known as methylxanthines, are found in coffee, tea, cola, chocolate, and medications that contain caffeine.

Fibrocystic breast disease is often a component of premenstrual syndrome (PMS). If you have symptoms of PMS as well as fibrocystic breasts, the treatment options in the entry on PMS may be more helpful. If fibrocystic breasts is your only or primary complaint, try the options below.

Most Helpful Supplements

- **Evening primrose oil:** may reduce the size of the cysts. Take 2 capsules three times daily.
- **Pyridoxine (vitamin B$_6$):** regulates fluid retention. Take 50 mg three times daily.
- **Vitamin E:** may resolve the disease. Take 1,000 IU daily of emulsion for one month.

Other Helpful Supplements

- **Acidophilus:** promotes the excretion of excess estrogen. Take 1 Tbs liquid extract, 1 or 2 capsules, tablets, or softgels; or 2 Tbs powder in cool liquid (not hot).
- **Chaste berry:** helps balance hormones. Take 40 drops liquid extract or one capsule daily in the morning.
- **Choline:** helps emulsify fats. Take 1,000 mg daily of phosphatidylcholine. See **lecithin.**
- **Dong quai:** helps balance hormones. Take 2 to 3 g capsules or tablets daily.

- **Germanium:** kills pain and promotes tissue oxygenation. Take 100 mg daily.

FIBROMYALGIA An estimated three to six million people, most of whom are women between the ages of twenty-five and forty-five, have fibromyalgia, which has uncertain causes and no known cure. The primary symptom is severe muscle pain, and it is usually accompanied by disturbed sleep patterns and/or insomnia and fatigue. Other symptoms include chronic headache, swollen lymph nodes, irritable bowel syndrome, swollen joints, numbness or a tingling sensation, and depression.

People with fibromyalgia have chronically low levels of the hormone serotonin. This deficiency causes the sensation of pain to be much exaggerated as well as the sleep problems that affect most people who have this disease. A magnesium deficiency is also associated with fibromyalgia. Stress exacerbates the pain, and low-impact exercise is recommended to help ease symptoms.

Most Helpful Supplements

Take 5-HTP, magnesium, and St. John's wort together

- **Cayenne (capsaicin):** relieves pain; apply lotion containing 0.025 to 0.075 percent capsaicin to affected areas.
- **5-HTP:** transforms into serotonin; 50 to 100 mg three times daily.
- **Magnesium:** may help relieve pain; 150 to 250 mg three times daily.
- **St. John's wort:** works in conjunction with 5-HTP and magnesium; 300 mg three times daily.

FLATULENCE Flatulence is the passing of an excessive amount of intestinal gas through the anus. Eating certain foods that ferment in the intestines, chewing inadequately, bacteria in the intestines, eating too fast, eating under stress, overeating, swallowing air, and constipation may all cause flatulence. Foods commonly likely to cause gas include beans, dairy products, fried foods, and glutenous grains. Beans and grains can be made more easily digestible if you soak them overnight and then cook them in fresh water. Foods to avoid if you are prone to flatulence include fried foods, sugar, hydrogenated fat (especially in snack junk foods), and very cold liquids. Combining spice or acidic foods with dairy products or sugary foods also can cause flatulence.

Most Helpful Supplements

- **Alfalfa:** contains chlorophyll, which aids in digestion. Drink up to 3 cups tea daily or take 1 tablet three times daily.
- **Ginger:** aids in digestion. Add $1\frac{1}{2}$ oz grated ginger root to 16 oz boiling water and let steep fifteen minutes. Drink 2 to 3 cups daily.
- **Goldenseal:** aids in digestion. Take 25 drops tincture three times daily.

GALLSTONES Gallstones are stonelike objects composed of various components of bile, a substance produced by the liver. The stones accumulate in the gallbladder and usually block the bile duct, which causes severe pain in the abdomen that radiates to the upper back. Nausea and vomiting also may accompany a gallbladder attack.

Gallstones may be composed of pure cholesterol; a mixture of cholesterol, bile salts, bile pigments, and inorganic calcium salts; pure calcium bilirubinate; or pure minerals. About 80 percent of gallstones in the United States are a mixture type. More than 300,000 gallbladders are removed each year because of gallstones.

Risk factors for the development of gallstones include a high-fat, high-cholesterol diet, obesity, sex (two to four times more common in women than in men), presence of gastrointestinal diseases, and use of some drugs, such as oral contraceptives and other estrogens. Prevention of gallstones includes eating a high-fiber, low-fat diet with little or no animal protein and eliminating food allergies. Fasting and rapid weight loss also increase the risk of developing gallstones.

Most Helpful Supplements

- **Choline:** protects against gallstone formation. Take 1,000 mg daily of phosphatidylcholine. See **lecithin.**
- **Milk thistle:** protects against gallstone formation. Take 600 mg (standardized to 70 to 80 percent silymarin content).
- **Peppermint:** helps dissolve gallstones. Take 1 to 2 capsules (0.2 mL oil per capsule) three times daily between meals.
- **Psyllium:** helps lower cholesterol levels. Take 5 g daily, in divided doses.

Other Helpful Supplements

- **Vitamin C:** a deficiency can cause gallstones. Take 500 to 1,000 mg three times daily.
- **Vitamin E:** prevents fats from becoming rancid; 200 to 400 IU daily.

GINGIVITIS Gingivitis is inflammation of the gums. It is a very common problem, and among people age thirty and older, it is a major cause of tooth loss. Nearly all people older than sixty have some degree of gingivitis.

Symptoms of gingivitis include swollen, reddened gums, bleeding gums, loose teeth, pain, and bad breath. The primary cause is poor dental hygiene, which allows the formation of a bacterial film called plaque along the gum line and between the teeth. Use of certain medications, vitamin deficiencies, and various medical conditions can make people more susceptible to gingivitis, but they are not the main cause. Individuals at high risk of developing gingivitis include smokers and those with Crohn's disease, diabetes, or leukemia.

Most Helpful Supplements

- **ACES:** promotes healing of gums. Take up to 250,000 IU beta-carotene daily for up to six months; 3,000–5,000 mg vitamin C daily; 400–800 IU vitamin E daily; and 400 mcg selenium daily.
- **Coenzyme Q10:** relieves symptoms. Take 50 mg daily for three weeks.
- **Goldenseal:** fights infection. Rub the powder on the gums.
- **Quercetin:** enhances the potency of vitamin C. Take 300 mg three times daily with vitamin C.

Other Helpful Supplements

- **Chamomile:** relieves inflammation. Drink up to 3 cups of the tea daily.
- **Folic acid:** reduces inflammation and bleeding. Rinse your mouth with 5 mL of a 0.1 percent solution of folic acid twice a day for thirty to sixty days; or take 4-mg capsules or tablets daily.
- **Green tea:** fights bacteria. Drink up to 5 cups tea daily, preferably with meals, or take 500-mg capsules daily.

- **Myrrh:** fights infection. Rub the powder on the gums.

GLAUCOMA Glaucoma is the presence of increased pressure within the eye (intraocular), caused by a buildup of fluid that cannot properly flow out. The improper flow of fluids appears to be caused by abnormalities in the structure of a protein called collagen in the eye. Stress also appears to be a major factor. Glaucoma affects approximately 2 million Americans and is the major cause of blindness among adults. Nearly two percent of people older than forty have glaucoma.

Glaucoma may be acute or chronic. Acute cases usually occur in one eye only and are accompanied by severe throbbing pain in the affected eye, blurred vision, a moderately dilated pupil, and nausea and vomiting. People with chronic glaucoma usually do not have any symptoms during the early part of the disease as the pressure increases slowly but persistently. Loss of vision is gradual and results in tunnel vision. Treatment of both types of glaucoma includes reducing the amount of pressure in the eye and improving the metabolism of collagen in the eye. Elimination of food allergies is often very helpful in people with chronic glaucoma.

Most Helpful Supplements

- **Ginkgo biloba:** reduces intraocular pressure. Take 40 to 80 mg three times daily of extract (24 percent ginkgo flavoglycosides).
- **Magnesium:** helps reduce intraocular pressure. Take 200 to 600 mg daily.
- **Vitamin C:** greatly reduces pressure; take as high a dosage as you can tolerate without diarrhea (see **vitamin C**). Suggested is 3,000 to 7,000 mg three times daily. "Vitamin C Flush," See p. 100.

Other Helpful Supplements

- **Bilberry:** assists in collagen metabolism. Take 240 to 480 mg daily in tablets or capsules standardized to 25 percent anthocyanosides.
- **Choline:** important when stress is a factor. Take 1,000 to 2,000 mg daily. See **lecithin.**
- **Chromium:** promotes health of eye muscles, especially in diabetics; 200 to 400 mcg daily.
- **Vitamin B complex:** important when stress is a factor. Take 50 mg three times daily with meals. Injections may be necessary in more severe cases.

GOUT Gout is a form of arthritis that is caused by an excessive amount of uric acid in the blood. Uric acid, which is necessary for the digestive process, is processed by the kidneys and eliminated in the urine. If the body fails to get rid of the excess acid or produces too much, it causes crystals to form in the joints and tendons, causing inflammation and pain. Approximately 90 percent of gout patients are men. About half of people with gout are obese and have high blood pressure.

Researchers have not identified the exact mechanism that causes gout to develop. Some theories include trauma, high levels of stress, adverse reactions to alcohol or drugs (especially antibiotics), and heredity. Symptoms include a sudden, intense pain in a joint, usually the big toe or ankle, accompanied by inflammation, a feeling of heat in the joint, and swelling. Poor diet is one of the main contributors to gout; thus attention to nutrition and supplements can be an effective treatment. Foods high in purines, which are needed to produce uric acid in the body, should be eliminated. These include meat, shellfish, fatty fish, asparagus, mushrooms, spinach, and dried beans. Alcohol should be avoided, because it hinders the elimination of uric acid.

Most Helpful Supplements

- **Folic acid:** aids in protein metabolism. Take 400 mcg daily.
- **Pantothenic acid (vitamin B$_5$):** antistress. Take 500 mg daily in divided doses.
- **Vitamin B complex:** antistress. Take 100 mg twice daily.
- **Vitamin C:** reduces uric acid levels. Take 3,000 to 5,000 mg daily in divided doses.

Other Helpful Supplements

- **Germanium:** helps pain and swelling. Take 100 mg twice daily.
- **Zinc:** aids in protein metabolism. Take 50 to 80 mg daily.

HEADACHE AND MIGRAINE Headache is a pain in the head that most often is associated with tension or stress, but can be caused by a wide variety of factors. Migraine is a very painful headache that sometimes also involves vomiting, problems with vision, and nausea. Headache and migraine are covered together because supplement treatments are similar and many of the triggers are the same.

Headache is characterized by a gradual increase in pressure and/or pain in the head, which may be mild, throbbing, dull, or sharp. Most headaches have more than one contributing factor. Tension headache is the most common type of head pain. It can be triggered by stress, eyestrain, too much noise or light, grinding of teeth, or poor posture, among other things. Typically the pain is dull and steady and feels as if there is a band squeezing the head. Often there is tension in the neck and shoulder muscles as well. A sinus headache is caused by congestion within the sinus cavities, which places pressure on the nerves in the face and head. Food allergies and ear infections also can trigger headache pain.

Another common headache type is the chronic daily headache. This type of head pain is actually caused by the medications people take to eliminate their pain—for example, aspirin, acetaminophen with or without caffeine or codeine, and ergotamine. Such drug-induced headaches should be suspected if you are experiencing headaches daily and take large quantities of analgesics.

Tension headache and the other types of head pain described above are examples of nonvascular headache. This means the pain does not come from changes in the vascular (blood-vessel) system, as do migraines. Migraine headaches are examples of vascular head pain. They appear to be caused by constriction and swelling of blood vessels and can be triggered by a wide variety of factors. These include but are not limited to food allergies or sensitivities, excessive use of caffeine, fluctuations in hormone levels (especially important in women), change in altitude or weather, low levels of serotonin, alcohol, chemicals (including MSG and nitrates found in processed meats), and eyestrain. When treating migraine it is important to identify the precipitating factors.

Migraines are characterized by pounding, sometimes debilitating pain on one side of the head, which may or may not be preceded by auras (visual disturbances), and is usually accompanied by nausea and vomiting. Common migraine, which makes up about 80 percent of migraine cases, occurs without auras and typically lasts one to three days. Classic migraine is preceded by visual disturbances and usually lasts several hours.

Most Helpful Supplements

- **Feverfew:** reduces frequency and intensity of attacks. Take a standardized extract that contains a minimum of 250 mcg parthenolide. Tincture—4 to 6 mL (1 to 1 1/2 tsp) three times daily. During a migraine attack, take 10 drops in water every fifteen minutes. Fluid extract—1 to 2 mL (1/4 to 1/2 tsp) three times daily. Take tablets and capsules according to package instructions. If using the dried bulk for tea, drink two or three cups daily.

- **Ginger:** antiinflammatory for migraine. Take 10 g daily. A fresh, 1/4-inch slice is the most effective form. Other forms include dried, 500 mg four times daily; or 100 to 200 mg extract standardized to contain 20 percent gingerole and shogaol, three times daily for prevention and 200 mg every two hours (up to six times daily) to treat acute migraine.

- **5-HTP:** raises serotonin levels. Take 100 to 200 mg three times daily.

- **Magnesium:** levels are low in both tension headache and migraines. Take 250 to 400 mg three times daily.

Other Helpful Supplements

- **Evening primrose oil:** dilates the blood vessels. Take 500-mg capsules two to three times daily.

- **Pyridoxine (vitamin B$_6$):** may help prevent migraine; 25 mg three times daily.

- **Skullcap:** for tension headache. Drink up to 3 cups of tea daily. The average dosage for the tincture is 20 drops twice daily. Skullcap is best taken after meals.

- **Valerian:** reduces stress. Make a decoction using 2 tsp dried root in 8 oz boiling water and simmer for ten minutes. Drink 1 cup daily as needed.

HEARTBURN Heartburn is a burning sensation in the chest behind the breastbone that occurs after eating. It may last for several minutes to a few hours and be accompanied by hydrochloric acid backing up into the throat, belching, and chest pain. The reflux of hydrochloric acid, which is used by the stomach during digestion, may be caused by spicy, fried, or fatty foods, coffee, citrus fruits, chocolate, tomatoes or tomato–based foods, or alcohol, or may be the result of ulcers, gallbladder problems, allergies, stress, hiatal hernia, or an enzyme deficiency.

In addition to attention to diet, avoid use of over-the-counter antacids, especially those that contain aluminum and sodium. Long-term use of antacids can cause a buildup of these substances and create a mineral imbalance or other problems. People with high blood pressure, for example, should avoid sodium products.

If symptoms of heartburn are accompanied by shortness of breath, dizziness, vomiting, diarrhea, severe abdominal pain, fever, sweating, or blood in the stool, it may signal a more serious condition, such as ulcers, hiatal hernia, gastritis, or it could be a heart attack. Seek medical help immediately.

Most Helpful Supplements

- **Ginger:** eases heartburn. Make a decoction by placing 2 tsp dried gingerroot in 8 oz boiling water and let steep ten minutes. Drink up to 2 cups per day.
- **Licorice:** eases symptoms. Take one 200- to 300-mg DGL chewable tablet three times daily before meals.
- **Peppermint:** eases heartburn. Drink up to 3 cups infusion daily, or take 2 to 3 capsules daily between meals.

Other Helpful Supplements

- **Aloe vera:** heals the intestinal tract. Take under guidance of a health-care professional.
- **Sulfur (MSM):** relieves symptoms. Take 3,000 mg daily for one week.

HEART CONDITIONS Heart problems, or cardiovascular disorders, are the number-one cause of death in the United States. Cardiovascular conditions include problems that affect the heart and blood vessels; for example, coronary heart disease, which is characterized by blockages in the coronary arteries, which in turn can result in angina pectoris or myocardial infarction (heart attack). Another type of heart condition is heart-valve disease, in which the valves that regulate blood flow in the heart malfunction. Some diseases in this category include rheumatic heart disease, endocarditis, and mitral valve prolapse. Pericardial diseases are those that affect the pericardium, which is the membrane that surrounds the heart. Primary myocardial diseases are those in which the heart muscle itself is diseased. Heart diseases that take shape in the womb are called congenital heart disease.

Each type of heart disease has its own symptoms, and most of the symptoms may also be associated with other medical conditions. Generally, angina pectoris and heart attack are characterized by a squeezing, suffocating chest pain that may last seconds or up to twenty minutes. Signs and symptoms of other heart problems may include swelling of the legs and ankles, shortness of breath, fainting spells, pounding or racing of the heart (palpitations), or sudden dizziness or light-headedness.

It has been proven that changes in diet and exercise habits can reverse heart disease in many cases. A low-fat, low-cholesterol, high-fiber diet accompanied by moderate exercise, no smoking, and stress management are key in the prevention and treatment of heart disease. Supplementation can be a major part of the program.

Most Helpful Supplements

- **Calcium:** aids function of heart muscle; 1,500 to 2,000 mg calcium chelate daily, after meals and at bedtime; take with magnesium.
- **Carnitine:** reduces fat and triglyceride levels in the blood. Take 500 mg two to three times daily on an empty stomach.
- **Coenzyme Q10:** oxygenizes the blood and improves exercise tolerance. Take 50 to 100 mg three times daily.
- **Garlic:** improves circulation. Take 2 capsules three times daily.
- **Lecithin:** emulsifies fat in the blood. Take 2 capsules or 1 Tbs with meals. Take with vitamin E.
- **Magnesium:** reduces the risk of arrhythmias and replaces magnesium depleted by drugs given for congestive heart failure. Take 750 to 1,000 mg daily (chelated to aspartate or citrate) along with calcium.

Other Helpful Supplements

- **Evening primrose oil:** helps prevent hardening of the arteries. Take two 500-mg capsules three times daily.
- **Germanium:** improves oxygenation. Take 200 mg daily.
- **Green tea:** lowers blood pressure and cholesterol. Drink up to 5 cups tea daily, preferably with meals, or take 500-mg capsules daily.
- **Hawthorn:** increases blood flow to heart, strengthens heart contractions. Take any of the following standardized formulas that contain either 2.2 percent

total flavonoid or 18.75 percent oligomeric procyanidins: 80- to 300-mg capsules twice daily; or 4 to 5
mL tincture three times daily; or 1 to 2 mL fluid
extract three times daily.
- **Vitamin E:** strengthens the immune system and
heart muscle. Take under a doctor's care—begin with
100 to 200 IU daily and gradually increase 100 IU
per week until you reach 800 to 1,000 IU daily.

HEMORRHOIDS Hemorrhoids are swollen veins that appear around the anus and occasionally extend out of the
rectum. Often they itch or bleed, causing pain, especially
when defecating. The most common causes of hemorrhoids are pregnancy, frequent or chronic constipation,
poor diet, lack of exercise, heavy lifting, obesity, allergies,
prolonged sitting, and liver damage. A natural approach to
preventing or coping with hemorrhoids is to eat a high-
fiber diet, drink at least eight glasses of water daily, and get
daily exercise, all of which will help avoid constipation and
keep the bowels clear.

Most Helpful Supplements

- **Calcium:** helps blood clotting and prevents cancer of
the colon. Take 1,500 mg daily. Take with 750 mg
magnesium.
- **Psyllium:** helps keep colon clear and relieves pres-
sure in the rectum. Take 7 g three times daily.
- **Vitamin C:** promotes healing and blood clotting.
Take 3,000 to 5,000 mg daily.
- **Vitamin E:** promotes healing and blood clotting.
Take 600 IU daily.

HERPES Herpes is a virus that has been classified into two
types: Type I, which causes skin eruptions and cold sores
around the mouth; and Type II, also known as genital her-

pes, which is transmitted sexually. Type II is the more prevalent infection. Once the virus enters the body, it remains throughout the individual's life and periodically becomes active and symptomatic. Among women the symptoms include the appearance of blisters around the clitoris, cervix, and rectum, and in the vagina, and a watery discharge from the urethra. Some women experience pain when urinating as well. Men experience blisters on the penis, scrotum, and groin, swollen lymph nodes in the groin, and pain when urinating. In both men and women the blisters erupt within several days of their appearance, leaving behind large, painful ulcers. The ulcers eventually dry up and heal. In some people the infection becomes severe and causes serious brain damage and inflammation of the liver. Babies can contract the disease at birth, which can result in brain damage, blindness, and death.

Because there is no cure for herpes, management includes keeping it under control and relieving symptoms. The disease is transmitted through sexual contact, and the first sores usually appear within two to seven days. Repeat outbreaks of the disease tend to be stimulated by stress, illness, and unknown factors.

The amino acid lysine appears to help keep the herpes virus at bay, while the amino acid arginine stimulates viral activity. Good food sources of lysine include kidney beans, lima beans, soybeans, split peas, corn, and potatoes. Arginine is found in chocolate, peanut butter, nuts, and seeds. Other foods believed to increase the chance of an outbreak include alcohol, sugar, refined carbohydrates, coffee, and processed foods.

Most Helpful Supplements

- **Vitamin A:** promotes healing and prevents spread of infection. Take 50,000 IU daily.

- **Vitamin B complex:** antistress. Take 50 mg up to three times daily.
- **Vitamin C:** antioxidant. Take 5,000 to 10,000 mg daily in divided doses.
- **Zinc:** Use lozenges for sores in and around the mouth; 50 to 100 mg daily in divided doses. Use the chelated form. Also zinc sulfate ointment to heal sores.

Other Helpful Supplements

- **Acidophilus:** prevents growth of harmful bacteria; 3 capsules daily on an empty stomach.
- **Garlic:** natural antibiotic; 3 tablets three times daily with meals.
- **Goldenseal:** fights infection. Take 2 capsules three times daily.
- **Licorice:** the lotion inactivates the herpesvirus. Apply the extract containing glycyrrhizin three to four times daily.

HIGH BLOOD PRESSURE When the blood presses against the walls of the blood vessels at a level that is greater than normal, it is known as hypertension, or high blood pressure. One of the main reasons the blood does this is that the arteries are clogged with cholesterol, forcing the heart to work harder and harder to pump the blood through narrow vessels, which in turn raises blood pressure. Other factors that can lead or contribute to hypertension include smoking, obesity, high salt intake, use of contraceptives, stress, and excessive intake of coffee or tea.

A normal blood-pressure reading is defined as 120/80. To determine blood pressure, the amount of pressure it takes to stop the flow of blood through the arteries is measured at two points during the heart's action: when the heart is beating (the systolic pressure, the first number) and when it's at rest between beats (the diastolic pressure, the second number). Blood pressure is measured with an instrument called a sphygmomanometer, and the numbers refer to the level to which a column of mercury rises at each pressure reading.

Approximately 40 million Americans have high blood pressure, which places them at risk for heart failure and stroke. High blood pressure is often seen in people who have diabetes, coronary heart disease, kidney problems, obesity, arteriosclerosis, and adrenal tumors. Many people with hypertension are unaware they have the disorder because they have no symptoms. Warning signs usually indicate advanced disease and include dizziness, headache, sweating, rapid pulse, shortness of breath, and visual disturbances.

Most Helpful Supplements

- **Calcium:** calcium deficiency is common in people with hypertension. Take 1,500 to 3,000 mg daily; take with 750 to 1,000 mg **magnesium.**
- **Coenzyme Q10:** reduces blood pressure and improves heart function. Take 100 mg daily.
- **Garlic:** lowers blood pressure. Take 2 capsules three times daily.
- **Vitamin C:** improves function of adrenal glands. Take 3,000 to 6,000 mg daily in divided doses.

Other Helpful Supplements

- **L-Carnitine:** helps prevent heart disease. Take 500 mg twice daily on an empty stomach.
- **Hawthorn:** lowers blood pressure. Check with your physician for dosage.
- **Potassium:** if taking diuretics or high-blood-pressure medication, take potassium. Take 99 mg daily.

- **Vitamin E:** improves heart function. Begin with 100 IU and increase by 100 IU each month up to 400 IU. Take as an emulsion if possible.

INFERTILITY (FEMALE AND MALE) Infertility is the inability to become pregnant after having unprotected sexual intercourse regularly during ovulation for a period of twelve months or more, or the inability to carry a pregnancy to full term. Responsibility for infertility is evenly divided between men and women: in 40 percent of cases the problem can be traced to the woman, in 40 percent it is associated with the man, and in 20 percent both contribute to the difficulty.

The most common causes of infertility among women are a failure to ovulate, which is often caused by a hormone imbalance; and a blocked passage of the egg from the ovary to the uterus, which is often associated with **endometriosis,** infection, or growths. Other causes include the sexually transmitted disease chlamydia, pelvic inflammatory disease, smoking, excessive consumption of caffeine, being overweight or underweight, and age (fertility decreases after age thirty-five). Occasionally an iron deficiency causes infertility in women. Before taking an iron supplement, however, an iron deficiency should be verified by a physician.

Among men the problem may be a low sperm count, low motility (sperm movement is impaired), malformed sperm, or blocked sperm ducts. Wearing tight underwear or pants may temporarily raise the temperature of the testicles, which reduces sperm production. In both men and women fertility can be adversely affected by depression, anxiety, or exposure to radiation, pesticides, or other environmental poisons.

Most Helpful Supplements

- **Chaste berry:** may be helpful in women who have high levels of the hormone prolactin and a shortened second half of the menstrual cycle. Take 40 drops extract in liquid in the morning; or 1 capsule in the morning.
- **Vitamin E:** helps balance hormone production in both men and women. Take 400 to 1,000 IU daily. Begin with 200 IU and increase slowly, about 100 IU per week.
- **Zinc:** may improve testosterone levels and sperm counts in men. Take 25 mg three times daily. If you take zinc for longer than one week, supplement with 2 mg copper daily.

Other Helpful Supplements

- **Carnitine:** for men, improves sperm count or mobility. Take 3 g daily for four months.
- **Iron:** for iron deficiency in women. Dosing should be supervised by a physician.
- **Vitamin B$_{12}$:** can increase sperm count in men. Injection is the preferred delivery system for this condition.

INFLAMMATORY BOWEL DISEASE Inflammatory bowel disease (IBD) is a broad term for several chronic inflammatory disorders that affect the intestinal tract. Crohn's disease and ulcerative colitis are the two main categories of IBD. All forms of IBD share the characteristic sign of recurrent inflammation of various portions of the intestines, although symptoms may differ. Causes for these diseases are unknown, although food allergies, heredity, infection, and antibiotic use appear to play a role.

Crohn's disease is an inflammatory condition that can

affect the entire digestive system, including the small and large intestines, stomach, esophagus, and mouth. The disease typically first strikes around age twenty and can recur every few months or stay dormant for years. Symptoms include diarrhea, cramps, lower right abdominal pain, loss of energy, weight loss, lack of appetite, fever, and malabsorption. Recurrent attacks weaken the intestines and can cause bowel function to worsen.

Ulcerative colitis is present when the lining of the colon is inflamed and marked with ulcers. The disease is usually limited to the colon. Symptoms include bloody diarrhea, cramps, fever, frequent need to defecate, and abdominal tenderness.

People with IBD often have deficiencies of iron, vitamin B_{12}, folic acid, magnesium, potassium, vitamin D, and zinc; less often low levels of vitamin K, copper, niacin, and vitamin E are seen. Correction of these deficiencies is important, especially in children with IBD, because many of them fail to grow properly. A high-potency multivitamin-mineral supplement is recommended as part of any treatment program. Any supplement program to treat IBD in children should be supervised by a physician.

Most Helpful Supplements

- **Acidophilus:** helps digestion. Take 2 to 3 billion live organisms daily (about 1 tsp powder or liquid in water twice daily).
- **Garlic:** promotes healing. Take 2 capsules with meals.
- **Vitamin C:** promotes healing. Take 3,000 to 8,000 mg daily.
- **Vitamin E:** promotes healing. Take 200 to 400 IU daily.

- **Zinc:** to replace deficiency and repair intestinal walls. Take 25 to 50 mg daily (take with 2 to 4 mg copper).

Other Helpful Supplements

- **Echinacea:** promotes immune function. Take 3 to 4 mL extract three times daily.
- **Folic acid:** restores low levels and repairs intestinal walls. Take 800 mcg daily.
- **Omega-3:** reduces inflammation. Take 1 Tbs flaxseed oil daily.
- **Vitamin B$_{12}$:** restores low levels and repairs intestinal walls. Take 800 mcg daily.

INSOMNIA Up to 30 percent of Americans have insomnia, which is defined as difficulty falling asleep and/or waking up frequently or early. Approximately ten million people take prescription drugs to help them sleep, while many more take over-the-counter sleep aids. One of the major problems with taking drugs to help you sleep is that long-term or chronic use of the sleeping pills causes addiction (in the case of drugs in the benzodiazepine class) and disturbing side effects, including abnormal sleep patterns, which actually make the insomnia worse.

Studies in sleep laboratories show that 50 percent of all cases of insomnia are caused by psychological factors, especially depression, anxiety, and tension. Other causes include use of drugs (including caffeine and alcohol), hypoglycemia (low blood sugar), changes in a person's environment, pain, restless legs syndrome (an uncontrollable urge to move the legs), and fear of sleep. Natural approaches to eliminating insomnia include getting enough exercise, avoiding foods, beverages, and drugs that contain caffeine, and practicing relaxation techniques.

Most Helpful Supplements

- **5-HTP:** induces sleep. Take 100 to 300 mg, or take melatonin—do not take both supplements.
- **Melatonin:** effective only if the body has a low level of melatonin; have levels verified before taking melatonin. Take 3 mg before retiring.
- **Skullcap:** causes drowsiness. Take 1 tsp in warm water before retiring.
- **Valerian:** a sedative and antihypertensive. Take any one of the following forty-five minutes before retiring: 2 to 3 g dried root in 8 oz boiling water as a decoction; 4 to 6 mL tincture; 1 to 2 mL fluid extract; 150 to 300 mg dry powdered extract.

Other Helpful Supplements

- **Niacin:** 100 mg before retiring. Reduce the dose if you experience flushing.
- **Pyridoxine (vitamin B$_6$):** helps reduce stress. Take 50 mg forty-five minutes before retiring.

IRRITABLE BOWEL SYNDROME Irritable bowel syndrome is a very common disorder that affects the large intestine and causes it to have irregular muscular contractions. This abnormal action prevents waste materials from moving efficiently through the intestines, leading to a buildup of toxins and causing bloating, gas, abdominal pain, and alternating diarrhea and constipation. People with irritable bowel syndrome also usually experience back pain and fatigue. Symptoms of the syndrome worsen in some women before and during their menstrual cycle.

Researchers have not determined the exact cause of irritable bowel syndrome, although food allergies and stress both appear to play a major role. Foods to avoid include meat and dairy products, spicy foods, fried foods, processed foods, sugar, coffee, alcohol, and soft drinks. Wheat and wheat products cause symptoms in some individuals. Recommended foods include vegetables, fruits, rye, brown rice, oatmeal, and barley, and foods made from these products.

Most Helpful Supplements

- **Acidophilus:** promotes digestion. Take 1 to 3 billion live organisms daily, which can be achieved by taking $1/2$ to 1 tsp powder or liquid daily, or capsules.
- **Alfalfa:** improves digestion and cleanses the blood. Take 1 tablet or 1 Tbs liquid three times daily.
- **Peppermint:** soothes the digestive tract, reduces gas production. If using capsules, take an enteric-coated form, one to two capsules three times daily between meals. Tincture—2 to 3 mL three times daily.

Other Helpful Supplements

- **Aloe vera:** cleanses the colon. Take $1/2$ cup juice three times daily.
- **Chamomile:** soothes and tones the digestive tract and helps ease alternating diarrhea and constipation. Take either preparation three times daily between meals: prepare an infusion using 2 to 3 g powdered chamomile in 8 oz boiling water or add 3 to 5 mL tincture to hot water.
- **Evening primrose oil:** for women who experience worsening symptoms before and during the menstrual period. Take capsules or tablets—3,000 to 6,000 mg primrose oil, which will supply 350 to 400 mg gamma-linolenic acid (GLA).

KIDNEY STONES Kidney stones are small, hard formations composed of crystals of mineral salts, with calcium oxalate being the main or only ingredient in up to 85 percent of stones. Other less common types of kidney stones are those made up of minerals other than calcium, and those made of uric acid. Kidney stones can become trapped along the urinary tract and cause intense pain. Individuals can have one or more kidney stones at a time.

Diet plays a primary role in causing kidney stones. People who have stones composed of calcium oxalate or who have a family history of kidney stones should avoid foods that contain oxalate. Foods that have the highest levels of oxalate include spinach, rhubarb, beet greens, chocolate, tea, peanuts, strawberries, almonds, and nuts. Caffeine causes the body to increase urinary calcium and thus should be avoided as well. Other foods that raise urinary calcium levels and are best avoided include meat, dairy, poultry, and fish. People who have stones composed of uric acid should avoid foods that contain purine, which include meat, shellfish, yeast, fish, spinach, asparagus, poultry, and mushrooms.

Habits that help prevent all types of kidney stones include drinking two quarts of water daily, avoiding soft drinks that contain phosphoric acid, and eating foods rich in fiber. Watermelon is a natural diuretic that dilutes the urine and thus helps prevent kidney stones. Eat watermelon often and alone, because combining it with other foods makes it turn sour in the body.

Most Helpful Supplements

- **Aloe vera:** helps reduce the growth rate of urinary crystals when taken at low doses. The dose of aloe vera for kidney stones varies per person but should be less than the amount you would use as a laxative. For example, $1/2$ cup aloe vera juice twice daily is a laxative dosage; for kidney stones, try $1/4$ cup twice daily. If you experience loose stools, reduce the dosage.

- **Magnesium:** reduces absorption of calcium. Take 500 mg daily, as magnesium oxide or magnesium chloride.
- **Pyridoxine (vitamin B₆):** when taken with magnesium it reduces oxalate levels. Take 100 mg twice daily.

Other Helpful Supplements

- **Glucosamine sulfate:** lowers oxalate levels. Take 60 mg daily.
- **Vitamin C:** acidifies urine, which prevents stone formation. Take 3,000 mg daily in divided doses.

LIVER PROBLEMS Problems with the liver result when this organ is prevented from doing its job, which is to detoxify the body. When toxins such as pesticides, pollutants, chemicals, drugs, and by-products of metabolism are not properly eliminated from the body, they can cause cirrhosis, jaundice, fatty liver, and hepatitis.

Cirrhosis is chronic inflammation of the liver, usually, but not always, caused by alcohol. The accumulation of toxins in the blood can lead to jaundice, which is characterized by a yellow or orange discoloration of the skin and eyes. Fatty liver is common among those who drink alcohol, including moderate drinkers. Hepatitis is a viral infection that causes inflammation of the liver. Of the three types of hepatitis, type A is the least serious and rarely causes long-term liver damage. Type B affects the most number of people and occasionally develops into cirrhosis or chronic hepatitis. Type C can be dangerous because the virus may lie dormant for more than a decade and cause no symptoms while the liver gradually deteriorates.

Most Helpful Supplements

- **Licorice:** protects the liver, enhances the immune system, and promotes flow of bile. Take any one of the following three times daily: 1 to 2 g powdered root, 2 to 4 mL fluid extract, or 250 to 500 mg dry powdered extract (5 percent glycyrrhetinic acid content).
- **Milk thistle:** a very strong protector of the liver that can reverse liver cell damage. For hepatitis, 140 to 210 mg silymarin three times daily, or 120 mg of silymarin phytosome two to three times daily between meals.
- **Vitamin B complex:** essential for liver function. Take 100 mg daily.
- **Vitamin B$_{12}$:** essential for liver function. Injections are preferred.

Other Helpful Supplements

- **L-Carnitine:** may be associated with a deficiency. Take 2 to 4 capsules or tablets daily thirty minutes before or after meals.
- **Coenzyme Q10:** fights viral infection. Take 60 mg daily.
- **Dandelion:** promotes the flow of bile. Take 5 to 10 mL root tincture three times daily.

MACULAR DEGENERATION Macular degeneration is a serious eye disorder in which the macula, a tiny portion of the retina in the back of the eye, deteriorates central vision while leaving peripheral vision intact. The damage to the retina can be caused by or associated with various factors, including smoking, sunlight, diabetes, high blood pressure, atherosclerosis, and heart disease.

Approximately 13 million Americans have macular degeneration in some stage of development. This visual disorder typically affects people older than fifty-five years, and the risk of getting this condition increases with age. Damage to the eye most often takes the form of deposits that build up under the macula or, less often, of an abnormal growth of blood vessels that leak fluid into the retina. Macular degeneration cannot be reversed, but it can be halted, and risk for the disorder can be greatly reduced. It's been shown, for example, that people who have high blood levels of antioxidants have a lower risk of developing macular degeneration.

Prevention and treatment of macular degeneration includes reducing the risk factors for atherosclerosis and maintaining a healthy, antioxidant-rich diet and supplement program. These steps protect against free-radical damage and improve the supply of oxygen and blood to the macula.

Most Helpful Supplements

- **ACES:** fights free-radical damage. Take all of the following daily: 25,000 IU beta-carotene; 1,000 mg vitamin C three times daily; 600–800 IU vitamin E; 200 mcg selenium.
- **Bilberry:** strengthens and reinforces the collagen in the retina. Take 240 to 480 mg extract in capsules or tablets standardized to 25 percent anthocyanosides daily.

  Ginkgo biloba: reduces risk of developing macular degeneration. Take 120 to 240 mg standardized extract daily or 0.5 mL tincture three times daily.

MENOPAUSE Menopause is the time when ovulation ceases and a woman's menstrual cycle stops, typically when she is in her late forties or early fifties. The entire menopausal period can last up to five years. It is characterized by a decrease in the level of several hormones, including estrogen. These hormonal changes often result in symptoms such as hot flashes, vaginal dryness, headache, heart palpitations, depression, irritability, and insomnia. An increased risk of heart disease and osteoporosis is also associated with menopause.

In addition to the supplements suggested below, certain foods that cause hot flashes and other symptoms should be avoided, including meat, dairy products, sugar, and caffeine. Routine exercise is encouraged both for physical health and as a stress reducer.

Most Helpful Supplements

- **Black cohosh:** contains phytoestrogens, which have weak estrogenic activity and thus relieve symptoms. Take 40 mg extract twice daily.
- **Chaste berry:** helps balance hormonal system. Take 500 to 1,000 mg daily of dried herb capsules, or 1 to 2 dropperfuls tincture daily.
- **Dong quai:** helps balance hormonal system. Take 3 to 4 g daily of the powdered root in capsules, tablets, or extract, or make into an infusion.
- **Vitamin E:** helps eliminate hot flashes. Take 400 to 1,600 IU daily. Increase the dosage by 100 IU per week until the hot flashes stop.

Other Helpful Supplements

- **Calcium:** helps relieve nervousness and irritability. Take 2,000 mg daily in divided doses with 1,000 mg **magnesium.**
- **Evening primrose oil:** relieves hot flashes and helps in the production of estrogen. Take 500 mg twice daily.

- **Lecithin:** aids in assimilation of vitamin E. Take 1 capsule or 1 Tbs before meals.

MULTIPLE SCLEROSIS Multiple sclerosis is a disease in which the myelin sheath that surrounds the nerve cells deteriorates, resulting in a loss of nerve function. Most cases appear in people between the ages of twenty and forty, and women are affected more often than are men. Its cause remains unknown, although there are many possible explanations.

One strong possible cause is that a viral infection causes damage to the myelin sheaths. Another is that multiple sclerosis is an autoimmune disease, which means the body essentially attacks itself. A high intake of dietary fat in the form of animal fat has been linked with the disease, as well as an inability of the body to detoxify free radicals. The dietary link is supported by the fact that people who live in higher latitudes (e.g., northern United States, Canada, northern Europe, Scandinavian countries), where people consume a high amount of meat and dairy products, have a higher incidence of the disease. Food allergies, especially to wheat gluten and milk, appear to play a role in the disease progression.

Natural approaches to treating multiple sclerosis include avoiding fatigue, wide changes in temperature, and stress; and consuming a low-fat diet with little or no animal fat. These measures, along with the supplement recommendations below, can be effective if begun during the earlier stages of the disease, but do not appear to have a significant impact once significant disability has occurred.

Most Helpful Supplements

- **ACES:** boosts the immune system. 15,000 IU; 3,000–5,000 mg in divided doses; 400 IU gradually increased by 100 IU per week to 1,800 IU; 150 to 300 mcg.

- **Coenzyme Q10:** improves oxygen use at the cellular level. Take 30 mg two to three times daily.
- **Pyridoxine (vitamin B₆):** boosts immune system. Take 100 mg three times daily.
- **Vitamin B₁₂:** boosts immune system. Take 100 mcg twice daily.

Other Helpful Supplements

- **Acidophilus:** restores beneficial bacteria. Take 1 tsp (about 3 billion live organisms) twice daily on an empty stomach.
- **Evening primrose oil:** helps with myelin development. Take 2 capsules three times daily.
- **Ginkgo biloba:** may improve nerve function and improves blood flow to the nervous system. Take 40 to 80 mg extract three times daily (24 percent ginkgo flavoglycosides).

NAUSEA/MORNING SICKNESS   Nausea, or feeling "sick to your stomach," is a common condition that can be caused by a variety of circumstances and conditions. People can become nauseous because they have food allergy, gallstones, migraine, gastritis, mononucleosis, flu, stomach ulcer, or diabetes, or because they are constipated. Nausea associated with motion sickness is often seen in both children and adults. Another form of nausea is morning sickness, which often occurs in women during their first three months of pregnancy. The cause of morning sickness is unknown.

The suggested supplements listed below can relieve or eliminate nausea; however, the cause also needs to be addressed to prevent recurrence.

Most Helpful Supplements

- **Alfalfa:** is a good source of vitamin K. It works only when taken with vitamin C. Take 5 mg daily.
- **Ginger:** relieves symptoms of nausea, motion sickness, and morning sickness. Take one of the following three to four times daily: 250-mg capsules or tablets; 1 cup ginger infusion (250 mg ginger powder in 8 oz boiling water); or 1.5 to 3 mL tincture. Take on an empty stomach.
- **Peppermint:** relieves nausea. Drink up to 3 cups of the tea daily.
- **Pyridoxine (vitamin B$_6$):** take at the first sign of morning sickness. Take 10 to 25 mg three times daily. For motion sickness, take 100 mg one hour before trip, followed by 100 mg two hours later.
- **Vitamin C:** Take 250 mg two to three times daily. Is effective only when taken with alfalfa.

OBESITY People are considered to be obese if they weigh 20 percent or more than the body weight that is normal for their age, height, and body frame. A more accurate way to determine obesity is to measure the percentage of body fat. Women whose body fat is greater than 30 percent and men with a percentage greater than 25 percent are considered to be obese. Approximately 33 percent of American adults and 20 percent of American children are obese.

Although obesity was once thought to be caused simply by overeating, researchers now know that it is a more complex issue. Several factors may contribute to any one person's being overweight, including lack of adequate physical activity, consuming a nutritionally poor diet, low serotonin levels in the brain, impaired metabolism, sensitivity to insulin, and heredity.

Being overweight increases the risk of stroke, heart disease, certain cancers, diabetes, gallstones, arthritis, and respiratory disorders. Excessive weight can contribute to infertility, osteoporosis, varicose veins, PMS symptoms, and hypertension. Many natural substances can help people lose weight; however, a healthy diet, regular exercise, and a positive attitude are the mainstays of a successful weight-loss program.

Most Helpful Supplements

- **Chromium:** increases fat metabolism. Take 200 to 400 mcg chromium picolinate.
- **Coenzyme Q10:** promotes weight loss. Take 100 to 300 mg daily.
- **Ephedra:** increases fat metabolism. Take 250 to 500 mg solid extract three times daily, or up to 2 cups daily of infusion prepared with 500 to 1,000 mg dried herb.
- **5-HTP:** increases serotonin levels, which reduces hunger. Take 100 mg 20 minutes before each meal for two weeks. If weight loss has been less than 1 pound per week, increase 5-HTP to 200 mg before each meal. Otherwise remain at 100 mg.

Other Helpful Supplements

- **L-Carnitine:** helps metabolize fat and reduce feelings of hunger. Take 1 to 3 g daily.
- **DHEA:** increases fat metabolism and converts fat to muscle. Take 30 to 90 mg daily.
- **Ginkgo biloba:** take 120 to 160 mg two or three times daily for tablets and capsules; 40 to 80 mg three times daily for extract.
- **Psyllium:** reduces fat absorption. Stir $1/2$ to 1 tsp psyllium powder or husks in 8 oz water and drink 2 cups per day. Do not take any other supplements or medications at the same time.

OSTEOARTHRITIS Osteoarthritis is a degenerative disease in which the cartilage at the ends of the joints wears down, which causes friction between the bones. Over time the ligaments, tendons, and muscles that hold the joints together become weaker and the joints then become stiff, deformed, and painful. More than 40 million Americans are believed to have osteoarthritis, and the chances of getting the disease increase dramatically with age.

Wear and tear on the joints places stress on the collagen matrix, which is the structure that supports the cartilage. As the cartilage is damaged, it releases enzymes that destroy the cartilage. The joints most often affected by osteoarthritis are those in the hands, feet, knees, spine, and hips. The first signs of osteoarthritis are usually joint stiffness when rising in the morning and pain in a joint that worsens the more it is moved. Inflammation is usually not present.

The good news about osteoarthritis is that disease progression can be stopped and even reversed. A combination of dietary efforts, natural supplementation, and exercise is usually effective. Dietary considerations include elimination of simple carbohydrates and nightshade vegetables (eggplant, tomatoes, peppers, potatoes, and tobacco) and emphasis on low-fat, high-fiber, and complex-carbohydrate foods. Exercise that improves strength without stressing the joints is recommended—for example, swimming, walking, and isometrics.

Most Helpful Supplements

There are a great number of natural remedies for osteoarthritis that have proved beneficial for many people. Therefore, the following list is longer than that for most other medical conditions in this book. They are offered with the understanding that if one does not work for you,

you have several other promising options from which to choose.

- **Boron:** needed for manufacture of normal cartilage. Take 6 mg daily.
- **Boswellia:** inhibits inflammation and promotes blood flow to the joints. Take 400 mg three times daily.
- **Calcium:** helps prevent bone loss. Take 2,000 mg daily along with 1,000 mg **magnesium.**
- **Glucosamine sulfate:** for pain and inflammation. If taking glucosamine alone, take one 500-mg capsule three times daily. For combination products dosage is dependent upon body weight. If you weigh less than 120 pounds, take 1,000 mg glucosamine and 800 mg chondroitin; 120 to 200 pounds, 1,500 mg glucosamine and 1,200 mg chondroitin; and more than 200 pounds, 2,000 mg glucosamine and 1,600 mg chondroitin.
- **Sulfur (MSM):** relieves inflammation and pain. Begin with 500 mg daily, gradually increasing by 500 mg every few days until you notice relief, or to a maximum of 5,000 mg daily.
- **Vitamin A:** needed for manufacture of normal cartilage. Take 5,000 IU daily.
- **Vitamin C:** promotes cartilage formation. Take 1,000 to 3,000 mg daily in divided doses.
- **Vitamin E:** inhibits breakdown of cartilage. Take 400 IU daily.

Other Helpful Supplements

- **Cayenne:** as a topical, relieves pain. Apply a menthol-based cream that contains 0.025 to 0.075 percent capsaicin up to four times daily.
- **Evening primrose oil:** controls inflammation and pain. Take 2 capsules twice daily.
- **Germanium:** relieves pain. Take 200 mg daily.
- **Niacinamide:** relieves pain and improves function. Take 500 mg six times daily. Liver enzyme levels must be checked every four to six months by your physician if you take this supplement.
- **Omega-3:** reduces inflammation. Take 1 Tbs flaxseed oil daily.

OSTEOPOROSIS Osteoporosis is the progressive loss of bone density, a condition that affects more than 20 million Americans. Women are at much greater risk for osteoporosis than are men because they have lower bone density before the age of forty. The group with the highest rate of osteoporosis is postmenopausal women.

Bone loss can occur throughout the body, but the areas typically most affected are the spine, hips, and ribs. More than 1.5 million fractures occur each year as a direct result of osteoporosis, with approximately 250,000 of these involving the hip. Hip fractures result in death in 12 to 20 percent of cases and in long-term nursing-home care for about 50 percent of those who survive.

Although many people believe a lack of dietary calcium is the only or primary cause of osteoporosis, several other factors are critical as well. More than two dozen nutrients are required for healthy bone, with calcium and vitamin D being the most important. Adequate absorption of calcium depends on a sufficient supply of stomach acid, which is lacking in about 40 percent of postmenopausal women. Another contributing factor is low levels of estrogen. As a woman's estrogen levels decline, there is an increase in the breakdown of bone and an increase in the amount of calcium excreted in the urine. Other risk factors for osteoporosis in women include excessive alcohol use, high intake of phosphates (found in soft drinks), hyperthyroidism, smoking, inactivity, family history of osteoporosis, and premature menopause.

Osteoporosis is very often preventable if a healthy diet and lifestyle habits are followed. The treatment options listed here are for both prevention of the disease and prevention of disease progression.

Most Helpful Supplements

- **Boron:** improves absorption of calcium. Take 3 to 5 mg daily as sodium tetrahydroborate.
- **Calcium:** necessary for bone formation. Take 1,500 to 2,000 mg daily, along with 750 to 1,000 mg **magnesium.**

Other Helpful Supplements

- **Manganese:** often low in people with osteoporosis. Take 10 to 50 mg daily with meals.
- **Phosphorus:** improves bone formation. Take 99 mg daily.
- **Vitamin D:** helpful for the elderly and people who do not get sufficient exposure to the sun. Take 400 IU daily.
- **Zinc:** improves calcium uptake. Take 50 mg daily.

PARKINSON'S DISEASE Parkinson's disease is a progressive degeneration of the nervous system, characterized by tremors (shaking), especially of the hands and face when at rest, a shuffling gait, trouble stopping or turning when walking, difficulty maintaining balance, and monotone speech. Symptoms and the rate of deterioration vary from person to person.

Parkinson's disease is caused by a deterioration of nerve cells deep in the brain in an area called the basal ganglia. The basal ganglia processes signals and messages via chemical neurotransmitters, the primary one of which is dopamine. Destruction of nerve cells in the basal ganglia results in a reduction in dopamine, which in turn reduces the number of signals and messages that get through. Scientists do not know what causes this destruction to occur.

Various drugs are used to help Parkinson's disease patients maintain as much mobility and independence as possible, including levodopa (the main treatment for Parkinson's disease) and carbidopa, and less often, selegiline, bromocriptine, or pergolide. For most people these drugs become less effective after they take them for several years.

Most Helpful Supplements

- **Calcium:** needed for nerve signal transmission. Take 1,500 mg, along with 750 mg **magnesium.**
- **Lecithin** (and/or phosphatidylcholine): needed for nerve signal transmission. Take 1 Tbs three times daily.
- **Pyridoxine (vitamin B$_6$):** production of dopamine depends on pyridoxine. Take up to 1,000 mg daily.
- **Vitamin B complex:** critical for brain function. Take 100 mg three times daily with meals.
- **Vitamin C:** antioxidants can slow progression of disease in people not yet taking medication. Also improves cerebral circulation. Take 3,000 to 8,000 mg daily in divided doses.
- **Vitamin E:** can slow progression of disease in people not yet taking medication. Begin with 200 IU daily

and gradually increase dosage by 100 IU per week until you reach 1,000 IU daily.

PMS Premenstrual syndrome is a combination of symptoms that occur seven to fourteen days before menstruation. An estimated 40 percent of women experience PMS each month. Symptoms may include and are not limited to fatigue, irritability, depression, headache, nervousness, anxiety, mood swings, abdominal bloating, diarrhea and/or constipation, cravings for sugar, tender and enlarged breasts, uterine cramping, altered sex drive, backache, acne, and swelling of the ankles and fingers. These symptoms are the result of fluctuations in a woman's hormone levels (estrogen and progesterone) prior to menstruation.

Most Helpful Supplements

The long list of effective options for PMS reflects the many symptoms associated with the syndrome. Choose the option(s) that matches your symptoms.

- **Black cohosh:** reduces cramping, depression, and mood swings. Take one 4-mg tablet (27-deoxyacteine) once or twice daily.
- **Calcium:** improves mood and reduces water retention. Take 1,000 mg daily in divided doses.
- **Magnesium:** helps relieve pain and nervousness. Take 12 mg per 2.2 pounds of body weight (e.g., a 110-pound woman would take 600 mg).
- **Pyridoxine (vitamin B$_6$):** relieves depression and helps magnesium enter the cells. Take 50 mg one to two times daily.
- **Vitamin E:** relieves breast tenderness, headache, fatigue, nervous tension. Take 400 IU daily.

Other Helpful Supplements

- **Chaste berry:** helps balance hormone levels. Take one 175- or 250-mg tablet or capsule daily, or 2 mL liquid extract daily.
- **Dandelion:** mild diuretic. Take 2 to 5 mL leaf tincture three times daily.
- **Dong quai:** relieves hot flashes and cramps. Begin taking any of the following remedies on day fourteen until menstruation begins, three times daily: 1 to 2 g powdered root as a tea; 4 mL tincture; or 1 mL fluid extract.
- **Evening primrose oil:** relieves cramps and other symptoms. Take 500 mg twice daily.
- **Licorice:** lowers estrogen and raises progesterone levels, reduces water retention. Take any of the following forms three times daily: 1 to 2 g powdered root as a tea, 4 mL fluid extract; or 250 to 500 mg solid dry extract.
- **Zinc:** needed for hormone health. Take 30 to 45 mg daily.

PROSTATE PROBLEMS As men age, many experience problems with the prostate, a walnut-sized gland located just below the bladder and which wraps around the urethra, the tube through which semen and urine leave the body. Because old prostate cells do not die off as fast as new ones are produced, nearly all prostates grow larger as men age. This enlargement causes the urethral opening to narrow and disrupt the flow of urine. The result is a nonmalignant condition, called benign prostate hyperplasia, that affects approximately 10 million men. If not treated, the urethra may eventually become blocked and cause kidney damage. Symptoms include increased urinary frequency, urgency, and a need to get up at night to urinate, reduced urinary flow, and difficulty emptying the bladder. Another prostate condition that often affects men is prostatitis, which is an infection or inflammation of the prostate. Symptoms include pain during urination, discharge from the penis, and fever. Prostatitis can affect men of any age.

Diet apparently has a significant role in maintaining prostate health. Men should keep their cholesterol levels below 200 mg/dL, avoid exposure to pesticides (in food and environmental sources), eliminate alcohol (especially beer), sugar, and caffeine from the diet, and supplement with zinc and essential fatty acids. Increased consumption of soy and soy-based foods decreases the risk of developing prostate cancer.

Most Helpful Supplements

- **Garlic:** a natural antibiotic. Take two 500-mg capsules three times daily.
- **Saw palmetto:** improves urinary flow and volume problems. Take 160 mg twice daily of extract standardized to 85 to 95 percent fatty acids and sterols.
- **Zinc:** reduces size of prostate and diminishes symptoms. A zinc deficiency has been linked to prostatitis. Take 45 to 60 mg daily.

Other Helpful Supplements

- **Bee pollen:** Take 6 tablets or 2 tsp raw bee pollen daily.
- **Nettle:** improves symptoms. Take 300 to 600 mg of the root extract daily.
- **Pyridoxine (vitamin B$_6$):** aids absorption of zinc. Take 50 mg daily.

PSORIASIS Four to six percent of people suffer with psoriasis, a skin disease characterized by a bordered rash or plaques covered with silver scales. Psoriasis affects men and women equally, but is much more common among whites than blacks and rarely affects Native Americans. The disease is caused by a defect in the skin cells, which causes them to reproduce much more rapidly than normal. The two substances responsible for controlling this cell activity are cyclic adenosine monophosphate (AMP) and cyclic guanidine monophosphate (GMP). High levels of GMP and low levels of AMP result in psoriasis.

Poor digestion or absorption of proteins and a diet low in fiber are typical of people with psoriasis. Foods that contain arachidonic acid (found solely in animal foods) should be avoided, and intake of omega-3 fatty acids should be increased. Alcohol can significantly worsen psoriasis and should be avoided as well. Healthy liver function is important in psoriasis, as the liver filters the blood, and psoriasis is characterized by an increased level of toxins in the bloodstream. If the liver is unable to properly filter and detoxify the blood, psoriasis worsens.

Most Helpful Supplements

- **Milk thistle:** improves liver function. Take 140 mg of standardized extract three times daily. The dosage for milk thistle bound to phosphatidylcholine is 100 to 200 mg twice daily.
- **Vitamin A:** vital for healthy skin. Begin with 100,000 IU for one month, then reduce to 50,000 IU daily. See "Possible Side Effects and Precautions" under **Vitamin A.**
- **Vitamin B complex:** antistress vitamins that also help maintain healthy skin. Take 50 mg three times daily.
- **Vitamin E:** 400 IU daily.

Other Helpful Supplements

- **Capsaicin:** reduces redness and scaling. Apply 0.025 percent cream four times daily. Relief is usually evident after three weeks of treatment.
- **Chromium:** increases sensitivity of receptors to insulin, a hormone that is typically high in people with psoriasis. Take 400 mcg daily.
- **Evening primrose oil:** helps prevent dryness. Take 1 capsule three times daily.
- **Omega-3:** nourishes skin. Take 1 Tbs flaxseed oil daily.
- **Vitamin C:** essential for healthy collagen and connective tissue. Take 2,000 to 10,000 mg daily in divided doses.

RAYNAUD'S DISEASE Raynaud's disease involves the constriction of the small arteries that supply the fingers and toes. These blood vessels become sensitive to cold and contract, resulting in hands and feet that are hypersensitive to the cold. Symptoms typically come on quickly and cause the fingers and toes to turn white or blue. Tissue damage occurs as ulcers form and the nails become susceptible to infection. Gangrene may result if proper circulation is not restored.

Most Helpful Supplements

- **Coenzyme Q10:** improves oxygen supply to tissues. Take 60 mg daily.
- **Inositol:** improves circulation and lowers cholesterol. Take 500 mg daily.
- **Lecithin:** lowers level of fat in the blood. Take 1 Tbs with meals.
- **Niacin:** improves circulation in the small arteries. Take 500 mg twice daily.

- **Vitamin B complex:** essential for metabolism of cholesterol and fats. Take 100 mg daily.

Other Helpful Supplements

- **Germanium:** improves oxygen flow to tissues and relieves discomfort. Take 200 mg daily.
- **Ginkgo biloba:** improves circulation. For tablets and capsules, take 120 to 160 mg two to three times daily; for extract, 40 to 80 mg three times daily. It takes at least two weeks before results are apparent.

RHEUMATOID ARTHRITIS Rheumatoid arthritis is a chronic inflammatory disease that affects between 1 and 3 percent of the population. It can involve the entire body, although the areas most often affected are the joints of the hands and feet, ankles, knees, and wrists. Symptoms may begin at any age, although the usual age of onset is between twenty and forty years. Several weeks before painful, swollen joints appear, many patients experience fatigue, weakness, joint stiffness, joint pain, and low-grade fever.

Rheumatoid arthritis is considered to be an autoimmune disease, which means the body attacks itself; in this case, substances called antibodies attack joint tissues. Researchers have not yet discovered the exact cause of this autoimmune response. They do know, however, that various genetic and environmental factors are involved in the disease process.

Most Helpful Supplements

- **Boswellia:** for inflammation. Take 150 mg three times daily.
- **Ginger:** antiinflammatory. Take 100 to 200 mg of ginger extract standardized to 20 percent gingerol and

shagaol, three times daily, or include 8 to 10 g fresh ginger into your daily diet.

- **Manganese:** replaces low levels characteristic of people with rheumatoid arthritis. Take 15 mg daily.
- **Sulfur MSM:** relieves inflammation and pain. Begin with 500 mg daily, gradually increasing by 500 mg every few days until you notice relief, or to a maximum of 5,000 mg daily.

Other Helpful Supplements

- **Capsaicin:** relieves pain. Apply 0.025 percent cream four times daily. Relief is evident after about 2 weeks of treatment.
- **Copper:** essential when taking zinc for an extended period of time. Take 1 mg daily.
- **DHEA:** low levels may predispose people to rheumatoid arthritis. Take 50 to 200 mg daily.
- **Niacinamide:** 500 mg four times daily. Check your liver enzyme levels every six months.
- **Selenium:** combines with vitamin E to help reduce levels of inflammatory prostaglandins. Take 200 mcg daily.
- **Vitamin E:** combines with selenium to help reduce levels of inflammatory prostaglandins. Take 400 to 800 IU daily.
- **Zinc:** antioxidant. Take 45 mg daily. Best results are with zinc picolinate or zinc citrate.

SEBORRHEIC DERMATITIS Seborrheic dermatitis (seborrhea) is a common skin disorder that is characterized by oily patches of skin that form crusts and scales. This skin problem occurs when the sebaceous glands, which secrete oil, malfunction. Seborrheic dermatitis has several forms, including nigra (dark-colored patches), sicca (dry with scales), facier (appears on the face), and rosacea (condition that first appears in middle age and often reappears).

The cause of seborrheic dermatitis is unknown. Possible causes include vitamin deficiency (vitamin A and/or vitamin B; biotin deficiency in infants), hormones, food allergies, emotional stress, heredity, and yeast infections. A deficiency of vitamin B_6 (pyridoxine), which can be caused by taking drugs (e.g., oral contraceptives, penicillamine, dopamine, hydralazine) and exposure to FD & C yellow #5 dye, is one probable cause. Because of the uncertain nature of this skin disorder, it is best to consult with a dermatologist before starting therapy.

Most Helpful Supplements

- **Biotin:** take if there is a deficiency. Consult with your physician before giving biotin to infants. The adult dosage is 30 to 100 mcg daily.
- **Evening primrose oil:** promotes healing. Take 2 g daily in divided doses.
- **Pyridoxine (vitamin B_6):** effective in the treatment of the sicca form of seborrhea. Use the topical ointment, 50 mg/g in a water-soluble base.
- **Vitamin B complex:** needed for protein metabolism and tissue repair. Take 50 mg three times daily.

Other Helpful Supplements

- **Vitamin A:** a deficiency may cause seborrhea. Take up to 50,000 IU. (See "Possible Side Effects and Precautions" under **vitamin A.**)
- **Vitamin E:** promotes healing. Take 400 to 800 IU daily.

SHINGLES Shingles (or herpes zoster) is an extremely painful condition that is caused by the same virus that causes chicken pox. The virus may lie dormant in the nerve ganglions in the spinal cord for decades until something triggers it—for example, exposure to chicken pox in later life, stress, cancer, use of anticancer drugs, and a weakened immune system.

An attack begins with several days of intense pain in selected areas followed by an eruption of painful, itchy blisters. After about seven to fourteen days the blisters become crusty and fall off. The pain may or may not continue once the blisters are gone. The elderly are more likely to experience continuing pain for months to years. This lingering pain, called postherpetic neuralgia, can be excruciating and very debilitating.

Most Helpful Supplements

- **Capsaicin:** Relieves pain. Apply 0.025 or 0.075 percent capsaicin ointment on affected areas as needed. Never apply to broken skin.
- **Vitamin B complex:** promotes healing. Take 100 mg three times daily.
- **Vitamin C:** helps destroy the virus. Take 2,000 mg twice daily.
- **Zinc:** enhances immune system. Take 80-mg tablets for one week, then switch to 50-mg lozenges.

Other Helpful Supplements

- **Aloe vera:** eases pain of blisters. Apply aloe vera sap directly on the blisters as needed.
- **Oats:** soothes the skin. Place 1 to 3 cups raw oats into a muslin bag and place the bag into hot bathwater. Soak in the bathwater for fifteen to twenty minutes. An alternative is to boil 1 pound shredded oat straw in 2 quarts of water for thirty minutes and then add the strained liquid to your bathwater.

- **Vitamin E:** helps prevent scarring. Take 400 to 800 IU daily. Vitamin E oil applied directly on the blisters is also helpful.

SINUSITIS Sinusitis is an infection and inflammation of the lining of the sinuses. This condition causes an overproduction of mucus, which in turn causes stuffiness, loss of ability to smell, facial pain, headache, and chest and ear infections. Although antibiotics may be necessary for severe infections, natural supplements are generally sufficient for mild to moderate attacks and also promote healing of more serious cases.

Sinusitis can be caused by a serious cold, irritating fumes, smoking, upper respiratory infections, nasal polyps, or allergies. More than 50 percent of sinusitis cases are associated with a bacterial infection. The presence of yellow or green mucus indicates an infection. If you experience swelling around the eyes, see your physician immediately, as it can lead to asthma, bronchitis, laryngitis, pneumonia, or other respiratory conditions.

Most Helpful Supplements

- **Echinacea:** fights infection. Take at the first sign of infection: 40 drops tincture every four hours.
- **Goldenseal:** fights infection. Take a standardized preparation: 2 to 4 mL ($^1/_2$ to 1 tsp) extract or 6 to 12 mL ($1^1/_2$ to 3 tsp) tincture three times daily. Do not take longer than one month.
- **Vitamin B complex:** fights infection. Take 125 to 150 mg twice daily.
- **Vitamin C:** enhances immune function and destroys viruses. Take 2,000 to 10,000 mg daily in divided doses.

Other Helpful Supplements

- **Bee pollen:** enhances immunity and promotes healing. Begin with half a tablet or capsule to see if you have an allergic reaction to the pollen. If not, gradually increase the amount, beginning at 250 mg daily to a maximum of 1,500 mg daily.
- **Beta-carotene:** improves immune function. Take 25,000 IU daily.
- **Bromelain:** liquefies and reduces the amount of bronchial secretions. Take 250 to 500 mg between meals.
- **Zinc:** enhances immune function. Take 20 to 30 mg daily.

ULCER (PEPTIC) Peptic ulcers are erosions of the stomach tissue (gastric ulcer) or the first section of the small intestine (duodenal ulcer). Duodenal ulcers are about five times more common than gastric ulcers and about four times more common in men than in women. About ten percent of adults in America will have a duodenal ulcer at some time in their life.

Ulcers occur when the lining of the stomach and duodenum is damaged. For many years the medical community believed that the acidic secretions of the stomach were responsible for causing ulcers. However, research now shows that a bacterium, *Helicobacter pylori,* is present in up to 100 percent of patients with duodenal ulcer and in up to 70 percent of those with gastric ulcer. Factors that predispose to infection by *H. pylori* include low levels of antioxidants in the stomach and intestinal linings and low gastric acid production. Smoking and the use of aspirin and other nonsteroidal antiinflammatory drugs are also associated with the formation of ulcers.

Symptoms of ulcer include abdominal discomfort (usually described as burning, gnawing, or cramplike) forty-five to sixty minutes after eating or during the night. This distress is relieved by food, antacids, or vomiting. The abdomen may be tender, and some patients have blood in their stool. Dietary remedies include eliminating milk and milk products from the diet, consuming foods high in fiber, and adding cabbage and other vegetable juices to the diet daily.

Most Helpful Supplements

- **Licorice:** heals peptic ulcer. For active cases, take two to four 380-mg chewable tablets of deglycyrrhizinated licorice (DGL) between meals. For maintenance, take one to two tablets twenty minutes before meals.
- **Psyllium:** supplemental fiber. Take as needed. Begin with $^1/_2$ tsp psyllium seeds or powder mixed in 8 oz cool liquid and drink 2 to 3 cups daily. Increase to 1 tsp per 8 oz after one or two days. Stir the mixture vigorously and drink it quickly, followed by additional water.
- **Vitamin A:** rebuilds antioxidant levels. Take 5,000 IU daily.
- **Zinc:** promotes healing. Take 20 to 30 mg daily.

Other Helpful Supplements

- **Aloe vera:** relieves pain and promotes healing. Drink 30 mL aloe gel or juice three times daily or take 50 to 200 mg of powder or powdered capsules.
- **Vitamin C:** Rebuilds antioxidant levels. Take 500 mg three times daily.
- **Vitamin E:** Rebuilds antioxidant levels. Take 100 IU three times daily.

URINARY-TRACT INFECTIONS Urinary-tract infections affect the bladder, urethra, and kidney. These infections are typically caused by bacteria that enter the bladder through the urethra (the tube that carries the urine) and travel to the bladder. The result is inflammation of the bladder, also known as cystitis. Kidney infections typically occur in people who are susceptible to bladder infections and usually are more serious than bladder infections. Kidney infections should not be self-treated; professional medical care is needed.

Cystitis occurs much more often in women than in men, primarily because women have a shorter urethra than do men, and the anus and vagina openings are close to the urethra opening, which allows bacteria easy access to the urethra. The bacteria that most often cause cystitis and kidney infections are *Escherichia coli,* which reside in the intestinal tract. Two sexually transmitted bacteria, *Mycoplasma* and *Chlamydia,* also cause cystitis. Urinary-tract infections can also result from use of a catheter (a tube inserted into the bladder to empty it).

Symptoms of urinary-tract infections include an urgent and frequent need to urinate. Urination is often painful and/or burns, and the urgency may persist even after emptying the bladder. The urine is often cloudy, with an unpleasant odor. Among the elderly, cystitis may also cause mental confusion and incontinence. Treatment that begins at the first sign of burning during urination can often eliminate the infection without further symptoms. If painful urination is accompanied by fever, chills, bloody urine, vomiting, or abdominal pain, get medical help immediately, as these are symptoms of kidney disease.

Most Helpful Supplements

- **Acidophilus:** restores the population of "good" bacteria in the intestinal tract. Take 2 capsules three times daily.

- **Beta-carotene:** helps fight infection. Take 200,000 IU daily.
- **Goldenseal:** prevents bacteria from adhering to the intestinal walls. Take any one of the following three times daily: 4 to 6 mL (1 to 1½ tsp) tincture; 250 to 500 mg of standardized root in capsules or tablets, or 0.5 to 2.0 mL (¼ to ½ tsp) fluid extract.
- **Uva ursi:** an antiinflammatory, antibacterial, and a diuretic. Take either of the following three times daily: 30 to 60 drops tincture in 8 oz water, or 0.5 to 2.0 mL (¼ to ½ tsp) fluid extract. For capsules, take up to nine 400- or 500-mg capsules daily.
- **Vitamin C:** acidifies the urine, which helps eliminate the bacteria. Take 4,000 to 5,000 mg daily in divided doses (500 mg every 2 hours is suggested). Some physicians recommend taking more than 5,000 mg, if tolerated, as lower amounts may not significantly acidify the urine. If you are also taking an antibiotic, check with your physician before taking vitamin C, as it may interfere with the effectiveness of the antibiotic.

Other Helpful Supplements

- **Nettle:** antiinflammatory. Steep 1 tsp dried, crushed nettle leaves or root in 8 oz boiling water. Allow the mixture to cool, and drink 1 tablespoon every hour up to 8 oz per day.
- **Zinc:** boosts immune system. Take 30 mg daily.

VAGINAL INFECTIONS Vaginal infections, or vaginitis, are the most common gynecological conditions. These conditions fall into three major categories: bacterial vaginosis, which is the most prevalent type; candidiasis, or yeast infection; and trichomoniasis, a sexually transmitted disease caused by a parasite. A fourth category is nonspecific vaginitis, which is usually caused by an organism called *Gardnerella vaginalis.*

Vaginosis is caused by bacteria that naturally reside in the vagina, but which can cause an infection when the vaginal environment changes. Factors that can prompt changes to occur include use of oral contraceptives or antibiotics, nutritional deficiencies, pregnancy, diabetes, or serious illness. If left untreated, vaginosis can develop into a more serious condition known as pelvic inflammatory disease, which can lead to infertility or problems with pregnancy.

Candidiasis is a fungal infection caused by an abundance of yeast cells. Symptoms include intense itching and/ or burning of the vaginal area, accompanied by a white, cottage cheese–like discharge from the vagina, and a red, inflamed vulva. Trichomoniasis is apparent by the heavy yellow-green discharge from the vagina, a fishy odor, and painful intercourse.

A dietary approach to vaginal infections includes eliminating refined and simple sugars, dairy products, and foods with a high level of yeast or mold. Foods high in antioxidants, such as fresh fruits and vegetables (avoid dried fruits and melons because of mold) should be a big part of the diet.

Most Helpful Supplements

- **Acidophilus:** restores "good" bacteria. Take 2 capsules three times daily with meals. You can also douche with acidophilus. Dissolve 1 billion organisms in 10 mL water at room temperature for the douche.
- **Coenzyme Q10:** potent antioxidant that fights infection. Take 30 to 150 mg daily.
- **Garlic:** fights fungal infections. Take 1 capsule with meals.

- **Vitamin B complex:** often deficient in women with vaginitis. Take 100 mg daily.

Other Helpful Supplements

- **Vitamin B$_{12}$:** for *Candida* infections, because this organism prevents absorption of nutrients from the intestinal tract. Dissolve 1 lozenge (2,000 mcg) under the tongue three times daily between meals.
- **Vitamin C:** enhances immune function. Take 2,000 to 5,000 mg daily in divided doses.
- **Vitamin E:** promotes vaginal healing. Take 400 IU daily.

VARICOSE VEINS Varicose veins are swollen, dilated veins that usually occur in the legs. Approximately 50 percent of middle-aged adults have varicose veins, which are often accompanied by nagging aches and pains, leg cramps, or feelings of heaviness in the legs. Some individuals also experience fluid retention, discoloration, and ulceration of the skin. **Hemorrhoids** are a type of varicose veins that occur in the rectum.

Varicose veins can be caused by a genetic weakness in the veins or their valves, by excessive pressure within the veins, standing for long periods of time, heavy lifting, veins or valves damaged by inflammation, structural defects in the vein walls, sitting for long periods of time with little or no movement, and crossing the legs. People with varicose veins have a poor ability to break down fibrin, a compound that clusters around varicose veins and forms hard lumps. Obesity and a low-fiber diet also contribute to varicose veins.

Most Helpful Supplements

- **Bromelain:** promotes breakdown of fibrin. Take 500 to 750 mg two to three times daily between meals.
- **Vitamin C:** promotes healthy veins. Take 500 to 3,000 mg daily in divided doses.
- **Vitamin E:** promotes healthy veins. Take 200 to 600 IU daily.
- **Zinc:** promotes healthy veins. Take 15 to 30 mg daily.

Other Helpful Supplement

- **Bilberry:** strengthens vein walls. Use the tea externally as a wash on the affected area, or take 240 to 480 mg per day of capsules standardized to provide 25 percent anthocyanosides.

PART III

YOUR OPTIMAL
SUPPLEMENT PROGRAM

Everyone needs a foundation on which to build a supplement program that fits his or her unique needs. A nutritional supplement program includes vitamins, minerals, and other nutrients taken to help support good health and to treat or prevent illness and disease. Supplements do not and cannot make up for a poor diet, lack of exercise, damaging lifestyle habits such as smoking or drug use, or a negative attitude. Therefore, although a supplement plan tailored to your specific needs can make a significant impact on your health, it is also essential that you address diet, exercise, and other lifestyle choices for overall success in health.

Physicians, researchers, and nutritionists do not always agree as to the best dosage of any given nutrient. One reason for their confusion is that although there is much we know about nutrients and how they work, there is just as much we do not know. Research is ongoing and guidelines have been established to help consumers choose the best nutritional program for themselves that they can.

This chapter offers you the information you need to choose your optimal supplement program. That program should include a basic multivitamin-mineral supplement plus, as needed, other supplements that address nutritional and dietary deficiencies, special dietary needs, chronic medical conditions such as diabetes, and temporary ailments such as colds and flu. The guidelines and questions and answers that make up the rest of this chapter are the tools you need to make your supplement selection and shopping effective and easy. And as a general rule, always consult with your health-care provider before beginning a supplement program.

How to Create Your Optimal Supplement Program

You can create your own program in three simple steps, which are listed here. An explanation of each step and examples of people who have done them are provided after the list.

1. Choose a high-quality multivitamin-mineral with the help of Table III-1 and the evaluation of your dietary habits.
2. Evaluate any additional nutritional needs with the help of the "People with Special Needs" and "Drugs That Cause Nutritional Deficiencies" sections and the "Supplement/Medical Conditions" charts at the beginning of this chapter.
3. Go shopping with a copy of Table III-1 and your list of additional supplements.

It's that easy. Now let's begin to decide your supplement needs.

CHOOSE A
MULTIVITAMIN-MINERAL

There are dozens of multivitamin-mineral supplements on the market claiming to be the one you need. Don't let the wide selection overwhelm you. Evaluate your dietary habits, refer to Table III-1, and you will have the information you need to choose the basic multivitamin-mineral that is right for you.

EVALUATE YOUR DIETARY HABITS If your dietary habits are good—for example, you eat mostly or all whole, natural foods; you consume at least five servings of fruits or vegetables daily; you drink pure water; your fat intake is less than 30 percent—a supplement with values at the lower end of the ranges is probably adequate for you. If, however, you eat lots of fast, processed foods, your idea of breakfast is a cup of coffee and a doughnut, and the last vegetable you remember eating was French fries, you need a supplement that contains nutrients at the high end (plus a new diet plan!).

For some nutrients, such as calcium, vitamin C, and vitamin E, you may need to take a separate supplement to get the recommended dosage for your needs, because many people do not get adequate levels of these nutrients in their diet, and multivitamin-minerals usually cannot provide the amounts most people need.

CHOOSING A MULTIVITAMIN-MINERAL SUPPLE-MENT A high-quality multivitamin-mineral is the base upon which you build the rest of your supplement program. Your chosen multiple should contain all of the vitamins and minerals as shown in Table III-1 and provide doses that fall within the dosage ranges listed. Some multiples contain minute amounts of trace minerals as well—for example, silica, vanadium, and iodine. These are not necessary, so do not worry if the supplement you choose does not have these ingredients.

Here are a few additional questions to consider when shopping for your multivitamin-mineral supplement.

What is a "high potency" supplement? Is more better?

"High potency," according to government regulations, means that the product contains 100 percent or more of the Daily Value (DV) for that particular nutrient. (See question about DVs in "Step Three" below.) If the product contains many nutrients—for example, a multivitamin-mineral supplement—at least two thirds of the nutrients must contribute more than 100 percent of the DVs to be classified as high potency.

More is not always better, and in some cases can be dangerous. According to *The Nutrition Desk Reference*, avoid any supplement that provides more than 300 percent of the DRIs for *all* the ingredients listed. Although it may sound like a good deal, such a supplement can upset the balance of nutrients in the body by providing excessive amounts of some in relation to others. Also, beware of nutrients you don't need. Do not take a multivitamin-mineral supple-

TABLE III-I

NUTRIENT	RECOMMENDED RANGE
Vitamins:	
Vitamin A (preferably all as beta-carotene)	5,000 IU★
Beta-carotene (if not as vitamin A)	5,000–25,000 IU
Vitamin B_1 (thiamin)	10–100 mg
Vitamin B_2 (riboflavin)	10–50 mg
Vitamin B_3 (niacin/niacinamide)	10–100/10–30 mg
Pantothenic acid (vitamin B_5)	25–100 mg
Vitamin B_6 (pyridoxine)	25–100 mg
Biotin (vitamin B_7)	100–300 mcg
Folic acid (vitamin B_9)	400 mcg†
Vitamin B_{12}	400 mcg
Vitamin C	100–1,000 mg
Vitamin D	100–400 IU
Vitamin E (d-alpha tocopherol)	100–800 IU
Choline	10–100 mg
Minerals	
Calcium	250–1,500 mg‡
Chromium	200–400 mcg
Copper	1–2 mg
Iron	15–30 mg§
Magnesium	250–500 mg
Manganese	10–15 mg
Molybdenum	10–25 mcg
Potassium	200–500 mg
Selenium	100–200 mcg
Zinc	15–45 mg

★ Women of childbearing age should limit their intake of vitamin A to 2,500 IU daily, as there is a risk of birth defects at higher amounts.

† Older people should take a supplement that contains 1 milligram, because higher amounts can hide a severe deficiency of vitamin B_{12}.

‡ Best to take as a separate supplement.

§ Postmenopausal women and men typically do not need additional iron. They should choose a multiple supplement without iron.

ment with iron, for example, unless your doctor has told you you need iron. If you are getting adequate iron from your diet and then take additional iron, you may experience diarrhea, stomach cramps, dizziness, headache, and increase your risk of cancer, cirrhosis, and heart attack. Also, why pay for supplements you don't need?

One-per-day or multiple dosing?

A one-per-day multivitamin-mineral supplement may be convenient, but is it the most effective form to take? Cramming all the high potency you need into one capsule or tablet is hard to do in a size that you can swallow, plus it gives your body a "peak" of nutrients rather than a more even dose throughout the day. Experts generally recommend choosing a supplement that requires you take two to six capsules or tablets daily. In this way the dose is spread out over the day and your body can assimilate the ingredients better. Also, take the multiple with meals. Multiples taken in between meals can cause stomach distress and are not as well absorbed.

"Fighting" nutrients?

Don't worry about "nutrient wars"—certain nutrients competing with each other for absorption—when taking a multiple. Although it's true that some nutrients do fight for absorption rights (e.g., copper and zinc), the benefits of multivitamin-minerals far outweigh the minor competition among nutrients.

Time-release or regular release?

Doctors and researchers are uncertain about whether time-release supplements are superior to those that are not. The only vitamin proven to be more effective when taken as a time-release formula is vitamin C, although researchers continue to study whether others fit into this category as well.

Calcium in a multivitamin-mineral?

Most multivitamin-minerals contain a very low percentage of calcium, and with good reason—the tablets or capsules would be too big for you to swallow if they contained more. To get additional calcium, you will need to take a separate calcium supplement (and don't forget to take magnesium too). Remember: the usual ratio recommended is two parts calcium to one part magnesium.

● = most helpful supplements for each condition
△ = other beneficial supplements

Supplement	Acne	AIDS	Allergy	Alzheimer's	Anemia	Atherosclerosis	Athlete's foot	Backache	Bronchitis	Bursitis	Cancer	Canker sores	Carpal tunnel	Cataracts	Chronic fatigue	Colds/flu	Constipation	Dandruff	Depression	Diabetes	Diarrhea	Diverticulitis	Ear infection	Eczema	Endometriosis	Erectile dys.	Fibrocystic breast	Fibromyalgia	Flatulence	Gallstones	Gingivitis	Glaucoma	Gout	Headache	Heartburn	Heart problems
Acidophilus							●					△			△						●	●					△									
Alfalfa																													●							
Aloe vera	△																●					●													△	
Astragalus											●				●	●																				
Bee pollen																									△											
Bilberry														●																		△				
Biotin																				△																
Black cohosh																																				
Boron																																				
Boswellia								●		●																										
Brewer's yeast																				△																
Bromelain								●		●			●																							
Calcium			●																									●								●
Cayenne																																				
Carnitine				●																																●
Chamomile																															△					
Chaste berry																											△									
Chromium																				△					●											

Coenzyme Q10

Copper

Dandelion

DHEA

Dong quai

Echinacea

Ephedra

Evening primrose

Fenugreek

Feverfew

Folic acid

Garlic

Germanium

Ginger

Ginkgo

Ginseng

Glucosamine

Goldenseal

Green tea

Hawthorn

5-HTP

If a nutrient typically found in a multivitamin-mineral is recommended as part of the remedy for a medical condition or ailment and the suggested dosage is within the range recommended in Table III-1, it is not included in the chart. If, however, the therapeutic dosage exceeds the range in the table, it has been included.

Legend: • = most helpful supplements for each condition   Δ = other beneficial supplements

Condition	Inositol	Iron	Lecithin	Licorice	Magnesium	Manganese	Melatonin	Milk thistle	Myrrh	Nettle	Niacin	Oats	Omega-3	Pantothenic acid	Peppermint	Phosphorus	Potassium	Psyllium
Heart problems			•		•													
Heartburn				•											•			
Headache					•										•			
Gout																		
Glaucoma			Δ															
Gingivitis									Δ									
Gallstones			•					•							•			•
Flatulence																		
Fibromyalgia																		
Fibrocystic breast			Δ															
Erectile dys.																		
Endometriosis		Δ																
Eczema			•										Δ					
Ear infection																		
Diverticulitis																		•
Diarrhea																		•
Diabetes	•					Δ												
Depression	Δ										Δ							
Dandruff																		
Constipation																		•
Colds/flu										Δ								
Chronic fatigue			Δ	•	Δ													
Cataracts																		
Carpal tunnel																		
Canker sores			•						•									
Cancer																		
Bursitis																		
Bronchitis																		
Backache				•														
Athlete's foot																		
Atherosclerosis	•												•					
Anemia		•																
Alzheimer's			Δ															
Allergy				•						•								
AIDS				Δ														
Acne			Δ															

Pyridoxine

Quercetin

Riboflavin

St. John's wort

Saw palmetto

Selenium

Skullcap

Sulfur

Tea tree oil

Thiamine

Uva ursi

Valerian

Vit. A/Beta-carotene

Vit. B complex

Vitamin B$_{12}$

Vitamin C

Vitamin D

Vitamin E

Yohimbé

Zinc

	Hemorrhoids	Herpes	High BP	Infertility	IBD	IBS	Insomnia	Kidney stones	Liver problems	Macular degen.	Menopause	Multiple sclerosis	Nausea	Obesity	Osteoarthritis	Osteoporosis	Parkinson's	PMS	Prostate problems	Psoriasis	Raynaud's	Rheum. arthritis	Seb. dermatitis	Shingles	Sinusitis	Ulcer	Urinary tract	Vaginitis	Varicose veins
Acidophilus		△			●	●						●															●	●	
Alfalfa													●																
Aloe vera						△																		△		△			
Astragalus																													
Bee pollen																			△						△				
Bilberry										●																			△
Biotin																													
Black cohosh											●																		
Boron															●	●													
Boswellia															●							●							
Brewer's yeast																													
Bromelain																													
Calcium			●								△				●	●	●	●											●
Carnitine			△	△					△					△															
Cayenne															△					△		△							
Chamomile						△																		●					
Chaste berry				●							●							△											
Chromium																													

● = most helpful supplements for each condition
△ = other beneficial supplements

Coenzyme Q10

Copper

Dandelion

DHEA

Dong quai

Echinacea

Ephedra

Evening primrose

Fenugreek

Feverfew

Folic acid

Garlic

Germanium

Ginger

Ginkgo

Ginseng

Glucosamine

Goldenseal

Green tea

Hawthorn

5-HTP

Inositol

Iron

Legend:
- • = most helpful supplements for each condition
- △ = other beneficial supplements

Supplement	Hemorrhoids	Herpes	High BP	Infertility	IBD	IBS	Insomnia	Kidney stones	Liver problems	Macular degen.	Menopause	Multiple sclerosis	Nausea	Obesity	Osteoarthritis	Osteoporosis	Parkinson's	PMS	Prostate problems	Psoriasis	Raynaud's	Rheum. arthritis	Seb. dermatitis	Shingles	Sinusitis	Ulcer	Urinary tract	Vaginitis	Varicose veins
Lecithin											△										•								
Licorice		△							•		△																		
Magnesium			•												•	•	•	•											
Manganese																△													
Melatonin							•																						
Milk thistle									•											•							△		
Myrrh																													
Nettle																			△	△	△								
Niacin															△														
Oats																													
Omega-3					△										△									△					
Pantothenic acid								•																					
Peppermint						•																							
Phosphorus																													
Potassium			△													△													
Psyllium	•													△												•			
Pyridoxine												•					•												
Quercetin																													

Riboflavin
St. John's wort
Saw palmetto
Selenium
Skullcap
Sulfur
Tea tree oil
Thiamine
Uva ursi
Valerian
Vit. A/Beta-carotene
Vit. B complex
Vitamin B$_{12}$
Vitamin C
Vitamin D
Vitamin E
Yohimbé
Zinc

INDIVIDUALIZE
YOUR PROGRAM

Step Two is the part where you make this supplement program yours and yours alone by choosing the unique combination of individual supplements and dosages that meet your specific needs. After you have created your supplement list, it will be unlike any program another book could give you, because it takes into account your health and your lifestyle—here and now. When your situation changes—for example, if you stop taking antibiotics, improve your diet, get the flu, quit smoking, become pregnant, or develop diabetes—you can turn to this book and easily adjust your supplement program.

To help you individualize your program, read the following two sections: "People with Special Nutritional Needs" and "Drugs That Cause Nutritional Deficiencies." If you fall into any one or more of the categories discussed—for example, if you are pregnant, are on a very low-calorie diet, are elderly, or are taking medication—you are encouraged to choose a multivitamin-mineral that contains the highest recommended dosages. That step may eliminate or reduce the need to purchase any additional supplements for your program.

People with Special Nutritional Needs

- People who cannot digest milk products (lactose intolerance) may need to take calcium supplements.
- Elderly people undergo some bodily changes that impact their nutritional requirements. Metabolism slows down, caloric needs decrease, and physical activity levels usually lessen, yet nutritional needs remain the same, and in some cases even increase. One example of an increased need for a nutrient is vitamin D. Aging skin loses some of its ability to produce and metabolize vitamin D, which means the need for the vitamin increases. Postmenopausal women have an increased need for calcium, and both men and women who are elderly often need additional B_6 and B_{12} vitamins to help the digestive process. An increased inability among older people to fight off infection increases their need for antioxidants.
- Strict vegetarians and others who for religious reasons do not eat eggs or dairy products may need to take additional vitamin D, B_{12}, and calcium. There are adequate non-animal foods, however, that supply these nutrients.
- Homebound individuals and people in nursing homes, regardless of their age, may need a vitamin D supplement because of insufficient exposure to the sun. This situation is of particular concern in high-latitude regions during the winter and spring months.
- Some vegetarians may need to take additional zinc and iron because these nutrients are more easily absorbed from animal products than from plants. Vegetarians who eat a varied diet that includes legumes usually get a sufficient amount of these nutrients.
- People on very low-calorie diets may need greater

amounts of all the vitamins and minerals, but especially vitamin E, calcium, iron, zinc, and vitamin B_6, because of their poor nutritional intake.

- Pregnant women need additional amounts of nearly all nutrients during pregnancy. In particular, vitamin B_6 is needed because the fetus draws this vitamin from the mother.

- Smokers, people who exercise strenuously, and individuals who are under a great deal of emotional or physical stress usually need additional amounts of antioxidants, especially vitamin C.

- People who drink a great deal of alcohol have difficulty absorbing and utilizing many nutrients, especially the B vitamins.

DRUGS THAT CAUSE NUTRITIONAL DEFICIENCIES Certain medications, prescription and over-the-counter, can cause significant nutritional deficiencies. You may be taking one or more of these drugs for a specific medical condition, to help you lose weight, or to increase muscle mass, and not realize the toll it is taking on your body. (Alcohol, nicotine, and caffeine are included in this table because many people tend to forget they are drugs.) If you are taking any of the drugs listed on page 209 in high doses or for an extended period of time, you may need to take a supplement of one or more of the nutrients mentioned, or choose a multivitamin-mineral that contains a high level of the nutrient you need. Make a note of the nutrient(s) you need.

SUPPLEMENTS FOR MEDICAL CONDITIONS AND AILMENTS Nearly everyone experiences annoying, painful, or even temporarily debilitating symptoms from time to time: a tension headache, occasional heartburn, or monthly menstrual cramps. Some people suffer with more serious

DRUG	NUTRIENT DEFICIENCY
Alcohol (including medications that contain alcohol; e.g., cough syrups and elixirs)	Vitamins A, B_1, B_2, biotin, choline, niacin, folic acid, magnesium
Antacids (containing aluminum and calcium)	Phosphorus, thiamin, iron
Anticoagulants (e.g., Coumadin)	Vitamins A and K
Antihistamines	Vitamin C
Barbiturates	Vitamins A, C, D, folic acid
Birth control pills and estrogen replacement	Folic acid, vitamin B_6
Caffeine	Vitamins B_1, inositol, biotin, calcium, iron, potassium, zinc, vitamin E, vitamin C, vitamin B_{12}
Cimetidine	Vitamin B_1
Diuretics (non–potassium sparing)	Potassium, magnesium, B complex
Isoniazid	Niacin, vitamin B_6
Laxatives	Calcium, phosphorus, vitamins A, D, E, K
Neomycin, cholestyramine	Vitamins A, D, E, K, B_{12}
Nicotine	Vitamins C, B_1, folic acid, calcium
Penicillin (in all forms)	Niacin, vitamins B_6, K
Seizure drugs and sedatives	Calcium, folic acid, vitamins D and K
Steroids	Vitamins B_6, C, and D
Tetracyclines	Vitamin K, calcium, magnesium, iron

medical conditions that impact their lives, sometimes for weeks or months, sometimes for the rest of their lives. Natural supplements can improve the quality of your life by easing pain, restoring vitality, improving immunity, or otherwise making each day a little better. To help you find the most effective supplements to remedy a medical condition or ailment that is affecting your life, look at the chart in front of this chapter.

1. Locate your condition across the horizontal listing and then trace your finger down the column beneath it.
2. Stop at each solid dot or open triangle and note the corresponding supplement on the left side of the chart. The solid dots indicate supplements that are generally most helpful for the condition; the open triangles indicate remedies that are also effective but usually less so than the others.
3. Turn to the medical condition in Part II and see which of the suggested supplements you may want to try. You can get additional information about each of the supplements in Part I.
4. Write down the supplement(s) and form(s) to buy.

SHOP FOR YOUR HEALTH-ENHANCING SUPPLEMENTS

The list of recommended supplements you have in your hand is unique because it takes into account your special needs, lifestyle, and current state of health. You may feel a little excited because you are finally taking control of your health. The last thing you need is to have that newly gained self-confidence begin to crumble because you are faced with words you don't understand—words like *chelated* and *USP* and *natural* on the labels of the supplements you came to buy. The following question-and-answer section will clear up any confusion and make those worries disappear.

Is there a difference between natural and synthetic supplements?

According to the U.S. Pharmacopeia there is no proof that natural vitamins are better than synthetic vitamins, with the exception of vitamin E. Some sources say that some forms of selenium, chromium, and beta-carotene also have superior natural forms. Natural vitamin E, identified as d-alpha tocopherol, is better absorbed by the body than the synthetic form. The natural forms of selenium, called

L-selenomethionine or selenium-rich yeast, and chromium, known as chromium-rich yeast, also are better absorbed by the body than their synthetic forms. Natural beta-carotene, derived from algae, contains many carotenes that the synthetic beta-carotene supplements do not. In all other cases the natural and synthetic forms of any given vitamin perform the same functions and do them equally well. All vitamin supplements must undergo a significant amount of chemical processing to make them into a tablet or capsule, whether they are "natural" or not. Natural vitamins are recommended, where applicable, in Part I.

There are so many different forms of supplements—tablets, capsules, softgels, sprays, tinctures, extracts, powders—how do I know which one to buy?

For any given supplement there is always at least one form that is more effective than the others. Under the "What to Buy" section for each supplement entry, the recommended forms are provided for you. These recommendations are based on the effectiveness of the form. Among herbs, for example, standardized forms are usually superior to all other forms. Solid extracts, fluid extracts, and tinctures are generally more potent than are powdered herbs, infusions, or decoctions. Capsules may contain standardized powder or another form of the herb, but need to state so on the label. Sprays (see question, p. 213) are relatively new to the market and tend to be more expensive, when comparing dose to dose, than other forms of the same supplement.

You should also consider your needs and lifestyle. Many people have difficulty swallowing tablets and capsules, especially the elderly and people with various medical conditions. Sprays, tinctures, extracts, and powders may be best in these cases. If the supplement you need is available in tablets and capsules only, ask your pharmacist or physician if breaking a tablet into halves or quarters or sprinkling the contents of a capsule into liquid will change the effectiveness of the supplement.

Sometimes it is simply a matter of convenience or preference. Some people prefer to add their supplements in tincture or extract form to a glass of juice in the morning and evening; others travel a lot and find that spray supplements are most convenient.

How effective are supplements that come in spray form?

According to the *Physicians' Desk Reference* vitamins and other supplements in spray form are very effective because they are readily absorbed through the mucous membranes of the mouth, where the capillaries are very close to the surface. Supplements taken as a pill, capsule, tincture, extract, powder, or tea are absorbed more slowly than are sprays, which enter the bloodstream immediately. One manufacturer reports that spray vitamins are nine times more effective than pills. Spray supplements also have another advantage: they do not contain fillers, colors, waxes, and binders used in pills and capsules, just 100 percent supplement.

Spray supplements have not yet entered mainstream use and are often difficult to find. Consequently they tend to be more expensive than other supplement forms.

Do herbal teas (infusions and decoctions) really have any therapeutic value?

Yes, but the extent of that value can depend on whether the dried herb is standardized, and on the purpose for which it is being used. A cup of peppermint infusion may be the perfect remedy for stomach distress, while an infusion of milk thistle would be less effective for treatment of liver disorders than the standardized tincture. Generally, infusions and decoctions are less potent than extracts and tinctures.

What does % *Daily Value* (*DV*) mean on supplement bottles?

The percentages next to various nutrients on supplement packaging reflect how much one serving (e.g., one tablet or three capsules) contributes to a 2,000-calorie diet. You may need more or less than 2,000 calories, depending on your age, sex, level of physical activity, lifestyle, and general state of health, so you will also need more or less than the 100 percent DV.

What are DRIs and how effective are they?

In 1997 the Food and Nutrition Board of the National Research Council created a new term to replace the RDA—Recommended Daily Allowance. *Dietary Reference Intakes,* or *DRIs,* is an umbrella phrase encompassing all the nutrients that have an assigned RDA, as well as all those experts believe are important but that have not yet been assigned RDA status. Nutrients in this latter category fit under another new category, *Adequate Intake,* or *AI.* It will take some time before the terminology is changed on packaging, as manufacturers have been given several years to make the switch.

The DRIs are based on sex and age and on the assumption that an individual is in good health. The dosages are specifically designed to reduce the risk of chronic disease and do not take into account factors that can increase a person's requirements for nutrients, such as inadequate diet, stress, environmental toxins, poor-quality food, drug and alcohol use, smoking, and poor hygiene. Thus most physicians and health professionals view DRIs as the absolute minimum levels for nutrients and routinely recommend higher dosages for optimal health.

Does it matter where I buy my supplements?

Generally, a health-food or vitamin store has a bigger, more diverse selection of supplements than does a drugstore. Health-food and vitamin stores are also more likely to carry brands that avoid the use of additives known as excipients: nonnutritional ingredients that hold the supplement together. Making purchases through the mail or over the Internet is safe *only* if you know exactly what you want and have already seen the product firsthand at a store and have read the label, or the content of the label is fully available for you to inspect in a catalog or on the Web site. Do not buy supplements over the telephone from solicitors.

Should I be concerned about the excipients used in supplements?

If you have a food allergy or food sensitivity, you need to be particularly aware of the fillers and other added ingredients in supplements. Look for products that say they are free of wheat, yeast, milk, salt, soy, corn, starch, and sugar. This statement is usually separate from any list of fillers, so check the label carefully. Typical fillers include talc, rice concentrate, cellulose, silica, and magnesium stearate.

Vegetarians who want to avoid all animal products need to check labels for gelatin, which is made from animals, unless the manufacturer has specified that the capsule is vegetable based. More and more supplements are available with nonanimal-based capsules and coatings.

What are antioxidants?

Antioxidants are nutrients that work to prevent or reduce the damage caused by unstable compounds called free radicals. Free radicals are molecules that are missing an electron. They are created by the body when it burns food for energy, but they also are produced under other conditions, such as when the body is exposed to toxic chemicals such as tobacco smoke and gasoline fumes, when you consume fatty foods, and when you are under emotional and physical stress. Free radicals attempt to balance their lack of an electron by stealing electrons from healthy molecules. This action can damage cells and tissues, break down the immune system, and ultimately lead to chronic disease. Researchers now know that free radicals are involved in more than fifty different diseases, and they play a critical role in aging.

The four antioxidants considered by many experts to be the most important are vitamins A (beta-carotene), C, and E, and the mineral selenium, often referred to collectively as ACES. Antioxidants are found primarily in fruits and vegetables, as well as whole grains, legumes, nuts, and seeds. They are a key factor in the prevention of many medical conditions and diseases, which is one reason why the National Cancer Institute recommends that people eat at least five servings of fruits and vegetables daily. However, fewer than 10 percent of people follow this advice.

What is a "standardized" extract?

Herbal supplements often are labeled as "standardized" extracts, or "guaranteed potency extract." This means that the extract is guaranteed to contain a predetermined, or standardized, level of active ingredients. Experts have determined that identifying an herb's level of active ingredients is the best way to judge its quality. Knowing the level of active components allows more accurate dosages to be made.

What are "chelated" minerals?

A chelated mineral, such as chromium picolinate, means that the mineral is bound to a protein molecule, which carries the mineral to the bloodstream. Many experts believe chelated minerals are better absorbed by the body, yet there is some debate over this idea. Chelated minerals also seem to cause less irritation to the intestines and stomach.

What does the "USP" mean on supplement packaging?

The United States Pharmacopeia, or USP, is an independent, nonprofit corporation that sets the standards of quality, purity, strength, packaging, and labeling for drugs and nutritional supplements in the United States. It has been in existence since 1820. Its governing board is composed of more than a hundred representatives from accredited U.S. colleges of medicine and pharmacy, national associations such as the American Medical Association and the National Association of Retail Druggists, and departments of the federal government, including the FDA.

Three Sample Supplement Programs

Let's look at the supplement plans for three different people. In each case the individual looked at his or her dietary habits, evaluated any special needs, and then chose a basic multivitamin-mineral along with needed supplements.

MELISSA Melissa is a thirty-year-old office manager with two children in elementary school. She admits her diet is far from perfect: no time for breakfast, coffee and sweets at the office, often fast food for lunch, but generally a balanced dinner. Melissa describes herself as "always on a diet" and a "light smoker." She needs a multivitamin-mineral with dosages near the high end of the range, especially vitamin E, vitamin B_6, zinc, and calcium because of her low nutritional intake, and vitamin C because of her smoking. Her physician checked her iron level and recommended the multiple contain 15 mg ferrous fumarate. Melissa choose a high-potency multiple, yet it had low levels of vitamins C (60 mg) and E (100 IU), and the minerals calcium and magnesium. And although she has no major medical complaints, Melissa says she "gets lots of colds" and is tired much of the time.

Taking all of these factors into account, and recommendations by her physician to improve her diet and quit smoking, Melissa added the following supplements to her high-potency multivitamin-mineral with iron: 1,000 mg calcium and 500 mg magnesium in a combination supplement; 200 IU vitamin E; because she smokes and gets many colds, 1,000 mg vitamin C three times daily, increasing to 1,500 mg three times a day as her body gets used to the high dosage.

To fight the cold she was experiencing at the time, she chose 4 mL echinacea tincture three times daily, 1,000 mg quercetin with each dose of vitamin C, and a 15-mg elemental zinc lozenge every three hours for three days, then one every four hours for another four days.

KATHRYN Kathryn is a sixty-three-year-old grandmother who works part-time in a bookstore. She began to develop osteoarthritis when she was in her early fifties, and several years later she changed her diet from the Standard American Diet to one that includes mostly organic foods, no meat, fish several times a week, and no sugar. Since then she has managed her arthritis with daily use of ibuprofen.

Kathryn's dietary habits are very good. Because of her age she needs some additional calcium and magnesium, vitamins B_6 and B_{12}, and vitamin D. She and her physician chose a high-potency multivitamin-mineral that has 50 mg vitamin B_6, 200 mcg vitamin B_{12}, and 400 IU vitamin D. They also selected a calcium-magnesium supplement— 2,000 mg calcium and 1,000 mg magnesium—because of her age and the fact she has osteoarthritis. To treat her arthritis Kathryn began to take glucosamine, 500 mg three times daily, plus 2 capsules of evening primrose oil twice daily. Because her multiple contained only 15 mg zinc and she needed 30 mg for her osteoporosis, she added a zinc supplement to her program.

THOMAS Forty-five-year-old Thomas is an executive with a large management firm. He routinely puts in twelve- to fourteen-hour days during the week, and on the weekends he likes to unwind with friends and play basketball and touch football. He shuns caffeine and has juice and toast for breakfast. Lunch is his biggest meal of the day, and he eats out, usually ordering fish or pasta. Dinners are generally takeout or a burger and a few beers on the way home. Thomas's "weekend warrior" games have left him with bursitis. He doesn't smoke, but on weekends he usually finishes a six-pack of beer.

Thomas needs a multivitamin-mineral that has dosages in the upper ranges, because his diet is poor and his stress level high. He and his doctor selected a high-potency multivitamin-mineral that contained 100 IU vitamin E, 100 mg vitamin C, 12.5 to 25 mg of the B vitamins, and 10,000 IU beta-carotene. Thomas and the doctor decided on a B-vitamin complex, 50 mg once daily for stress and because of the toll alcohol takes on B vitamins; 1,000 mg vitamin C three times daily for stress and building tissue for treatment of bursitis; 300 IU vitamin E daily for stress and tissue healing for bursitis; and 500 mg bromelain three times daily between meals as needed for inflammation associated with bursitis.

Your Plan

Now it's time for your ideal supplement plan. Take the steps; consult with your health-care practitioner. Consider lifestyle changes as needed. And then prepare yourself for better health, vitality, and well-being.

GLOSSARY

Adaptogen. A substance that helps balance bodily functions and increases the body's resistance to stress.

Alkaloids. Natural nitrogen-containing compounds, known as amines, which have some pharmacological effect.

Antacid. A substance that neutralizes excess acid in the stomach.

Antibody. A protein, produced by the body, that helps fight infection by attaching itself to harmful substances known collectively as antigens.

Anticoagulant. A medicine that prevents the formation of blood clots.

Antigen. A substance that causes antibodies to form in an effort to neutralize, stop, or destroy it.

Antihistamine. A medicine used to prevent the action of histamines, which cause symptoms of allergy.

Antiinflammatory. A medicine used to relieve the symptoms of inflammation, such as pain and swelling.

Antioxidant. A compound that prevents damage from oxidation or from molecules known as free radicals. Antioxidants give an electron to free radicals.

ATP (adenosine triphosphate). A compound that is the main energy source for the body. It consists of one molecule each of adenine and ribose and three of phosphoric acid.

Beta-carotene. Also known as provitamin A, this plant pigment is converted into two vitamin A molecules.

Bioavailability. A measure of how available a nutrient or other substance is to the body once it enters the body.

Bioflavonoids. Compounds found in fruits that contain vitamin C. Some experts believe they should be given vitamin status.

Carotenes/Carotenoids. Fat-soluble pigments, found in plants, which the body can convert into vitamin A.

Chelated. When minerals are bound to proteins in order to increase their bioavailability.

Cholesterol. A fatlike substance that is present in the body from two sources: production by the liver, and what is absorbed from eating animal products.

Cirrhosis. A severe liver disease in which nonfunctioning scar tissue replaces normal liver tissue.

Coenzyme. An essential component of an enzyme, which takes part in the body's chemical processes. Vitamins and minerals are examples of coenzymes.

Colitis. Inflammation of the colon.

Collagen. The protein that is the main component of connective tissue.

Congestive heart failure. The result of the heart's inability to pump with enough strength to maintain sufficient blood flow. The result is shortness of breath, fatigue, and swelling.

Connective tissue. The kind of tissue that provides the body with structure and support, including the skin, muscles, blood vessels, bone, and gums.

Corticosteroids. Hormones secreted by the adrenal cortex (in the brain) that are involved in metabolism and the balance of salt and water in the body.

Cystitis. Inflammation of the bladder lining.

Daily Value (DV). A term that replaces the RDA—Recommended Dietary Allowance—on food and supplement labels. It indicates the percentage of the recommended daily amount each serving or dose provides.

Dermatitis. Inflammation of the skin.

Dietary Reference Intake (DRI). An umbrella term that includes the RDA as well as a new designation, Adequate Intake (AI). The DRIs are the daily nutrient recommendations based on sex and age and are designed to reduce the risk of specific diseases and medical conditions.

Diuretic. A substance that causes the kidneys to produce an increased amount of urine.

Douche. A method of introducing a cleansing substance into the vagina.

Eicosapentaenoic acid (EPA). A type of omega-3 fatty acid.

Emulsion. A liquid in which the fat particles are uniformly distributed. Sometimes used for the fat-soluble vitamins A and E.

Enteric-coated. A capsule or tablet coated with a substance that allows the capsule or tablet to reach the intestines before it dissolves and releases its ingredients.

Essential fatty acids. The two fatty acids—linoleic and linolenic—which the body needs but cannot manufacture. They must be obtained through diet.

Extracts. The concentrated form of herbs and other natural substances, available as fluid extracts, solid extracts, powdered extracts, and tinctures. Extracts are made by treating the natural substance with a solvent and then removing the solvent, either completely or partially.

Fat-soluble vitamins. Vitamins that are stored in fat tissue and can be dissolved in fat. They include vitamins A, D, E, and K.

Flavonoid. An umbrella term for natural compounds that contain flavones. Among flavonoids are many plant pigments, including anthocyanins, flavones, bioflavonols, and so on.

Fluid extract. Herbal extracts that typically have a ratio of one part herb to one part alcohol, water, or a combination of the two.

Free radicals. Molecules that have unpaired electrons and thus attach themselves to other molecules, take their electrons, and cause cellular damage in the process. Antioxidants donate an electron, which neutralizes free radicals.

Glucose. A type of sugar, called a monosaccharide, that is an essential energy source for the body.

Histamine. A chemical released in high amounts during an allergic reaction.

Hormone. A substance, produced in a gland or organ, that travels to other parts of the body to carry out specific functions.

Insulin. A hormone produced and secreted by the pancreas. Insulin helps carry glucose into the cells for energy and to the liver and muscles for storage.

Keratin. A type of protein found in skin, nails, and hair.

Lactose. A type of sugar found in milk.

Laxative. A substance that stimulates elimination of material from the bowels.

Malabsorption. An inability to properly and sufficiently absorb nutrients.

Metabolism. A general term for all the chemical processes in the body.

Mineral. A nonorganic compound whose origin is not from living organisms and which is necessary for the body's functions.

Monosaccharide. A simple sugar; for example, glucose or fructose.

Mucous membrane. The soft tissue that lines many of the channels and cavities in the body, including the mouth, gastrointestinal tract, and urinary tract.

Neurotransmitters. Chemicals produced by the brain and nerves that transmit and modify nerve signals and allow people to think, act, and feel.

Powdered extract. A solid extract that has been ground into a powder, which can be added to capsules or mixed with a liquid for easy administration.

Prostaglandins. Hormonelike substances, manufactured from essential fatty acids, which can cause inflammation.

Recommended Dietary Allowance (RDA). A designation

established by the Food and Nutrition Board of the National Academy of Sciences/National Research Council. The RDA was replaced by the DRI—Dietary Reference Intake—in 1997.

Retinol equivalents (RE). Units of measure used to compare and convert the different forms of vitamin A, because each form (preformed vitamin A, beta-carotene, and other carotenoids) has a different level of activity in the body.

Serotonin. A chemical produced in the brain that regulates many functions, including mood and feeling full after eating, among others.

Solid extract. An extract from which all the moisture and solvent have been removed.

Sublingual. A method of taking a supplement or medication by placing it under the tongue and allowing it to dissolve slowly.

Vitamin. An organic compound the body needs in small amounts to conduct normal bodily functions.

Vitiligo. A skin condition in which some areas lose pigment and turn white.

Water-soluble vitamins. Vitamins that dissolve in water and must be replaced daily because the body does not store them. They include vitamin C and the B vitamins.

APPENDIX A

SUGGESTED READINGS

Balch, James F., and Phyllis A. Balch. *Prescription for Nutritional Healing*. Garden City Park, NY: Avery Publishing Group, 1990.

Castleman, Michael. *The Healing Herbs*. Emmaus, PA: Rodale Press, 1991.

Cooper, Kenneth H. *Dr. Kenneth H. Cooper's Antioxidant Revolution*. Nashville, TN: Thomas Nelson Publishers, 1994.

Foster, Steven. *An Illustrated Guide. 101 Medicinal Herbs*.Loveland, CO: Interweave Press, 1998.

Garrison, Robert, Jr., and Elizabeth Somer. *The Nutrition Desk Reference*. New Canaan, CT: Keats Publishing Co., 1997.

Gottlieb, Bill, ed. *New Choices in Natural Healing*.Emmaus, PA: Rodale Press, 1995.

Klaper, Michael. *Vegan Nutrition Pure and Simple*. Maui, HI: Gentle World, 1987.

Mayell, Mark. *Off-the-Shelf Natural Health: How to Use Herbs and Nutrients to Stay Well*. New York: Bantam Books, 1995.

Merck Manual of Medical Information (Home Edition). Whitehouse Station, NJ: Merck Research Laboratories, 1997.

Mindell, Earl. *Earl Mindell's Herb Bible*. New York: Simon & Schuster, 1992.

————. *Earl Mindell's Vitamin Bible*. New York: Warner Books, 1991.

Murray, Michael T., ND. *Encyclopedia of Natural Medicine*.Rocklin, CA: Prima Publishing, 1998.

————. *Encyclopedia of Nutritional Supplements*. Rocklin, CA: Prima Publishing, 1996.

————. *The Healing Power of Herbs*. 2nd ed. Rocklin, CA: Prima Publishing, 1995.

The PDR Family Guide to Nutrition and Health. Montvale, NJ: Medical Economics, 1998.

Robbins, John. *Diet for a New America: How Your Food Choices Affect Your Health, Happiness, and the Future of Life on Earth*.Walpole, NH: Stillpoint Publishing, 1987.

Tyler, Varro E. *Herbs of Choice: The Therapeutic Use of Phytochemicals*. New York: Pharmaceutical Products Press, 1994.

U.S. Pharmacopeia. *Guide to Vitamins and Minerals*.New York: Avon Books, 1996.

Van Straten, Michael. *Home Remedies*. New York: Marlowe & Co., 1998.

Walker, Lynne Paige, and Ellen Hodgson Brown. *The Alternative Pharmacy*. Paramus, NJ: Prentice Hall, 1998.

Webb, Marcus A. *The Herbal Companion*. Allentown, PA: People's Medical Society, 1997.

Weil, Andrew. *Natural Health, Natural Medicine*. Boston: Houghton Mifflin, 1990.

Whitaker, Julian. *Dr. Whitaker's Guide to Natural Healing*.Rocklin, CA: Prima Publishing, 1995.

APPENDIX B

RESOURCES

For questions about supplements, nutrition, and health, contact the following organizations.

American Botanical Council
PO Box 144345
Austin TX 78714–4345
.1–512–331–8868

American Dietetic Association
216 W. Jackson Blvd.
Chicago IL 60606–6995
1–312–899–0040
http://www.eatright.org

American Herb Association
PO Box 1673
Nevada City CA 95959
1–916–265–9552 (fax)

Center for Science in the Public Interest
1875 Connecticut Ave., NW, Suite 300

Washington DC 20009–5728
1–202–332–9110

Food and Drug Administration
5600 Fishers Lane, HFE 88
Rockville MD 20857
1–888–463–6332
(or see the Yellow Pages for your regional FDA office)
http://www.fda.gov

The Herb Research Foundation
1007 Pearl St. #200
Boulder CO 80302
1–303–449–2265

The Kellen Company
International Food Additives Council
5775 Peachtree-Dunwoody Rd., Suite 500-G
Atlanta GA 30342
1–404–252–3663

National Academy of Sciences/Food and Nutrition Board
2101 Constitution Ave., NW
Washington DC 20418
1–202–334–1732

North American Vegetarian Society
PO Box 72
Dolgeville NY 13329
1-518–568–7970

Vegetarian Resource Group
PO Box 1463
Baltimore MD 21203
1-410–366–VEGE
http://www.vrg.org

PUBLICATIONS

Environmental Nutrition
52 Riverside Dr., Suite 15-A
New York NY 10024–6599
E-mail: 76521.2250@compuserve.com

FDA Consumer
PO Box 371954
Pittsburgh PA 15250–7954

Good Medicine
PO Box 420 235
Palm Coast FL 32142

Tufts University Health and Nutrition Letter
50 Broadway
15th floor
New York NY 10004

APPENDIX C

ADDITIVES IN SUPPLEMENTS

The next time you buy a supplement, you may get more than you think you paid for, and you may not be too pleased with the extras. Fillers, binders, lubricants, colors, coating material, and drying agents are the not-so-appealing categories of additives that are in many supplements on the market, and sometimes they are not even listed on the label. Here's a rundown of what you may or may not see on the label and what it means.

- **Fillers.** These inert ingredients are added to tablets to increase their bulk, which makes it easier to compress them during the manufacturing process. Better-quality supplements may use dicalcium phosphate as a filler, which also serves as an excellent source of calcium and phosphorus. Other fillers you may see in less expensive supplements are cellulose (plant fiber) and sorbitol.
- **Drying Agents.** These additives prevent the supplement materials from absorbing moisture during manufacturing. The most common drying agent is silica gel.
- **Binders.** These substances are the "glue" that holds the ingredients of tablets together. Binders considered to be safe include cellulose, ethyl cellulose, sorbitol, and lecithin. Binders that may cause a reaction in some individuals in-

clude alginic acid and sodium alginate, which are derived from seaweed and may cause reproductive problems and birth defects. Another is acacia (gum arabic), a vegetable gum that can cause asthma attacks and rash in pregnant women, people who have asthma, and anyone susceptible to allergies.

- **Lubricants.** Substances such as calcium stearate, silica, and magnesium stearate are used as nonsticking agents during manufacturing to prevent tablets from sticking to the machine that punches them out.
- **Coating Material.** Zein is one of the most widely used coating substances. This corn protein derivative protects tablets from moisture, makes tablets easier to swallow, and can also mask unpleasant odors or flavors. A derivative from palm trees, Brazil wax, is also sometimes used.
- **Color, Flavors.** Color is used to make tablets more visually appealing. Chewable tablets may contain fructose, malt dextrins, sorbitol, maltose, or sucrose as a sweetener.

WEIGHTS AND MEASURES

The U.S. measurement system is less accurate than the metric system when dealing with small measures. The following conversions are a rough translation of metric to U.S. measures.

Fluid Measures
    1 mL = 10 drops = 1/5 tsp
    5 mL = 50 drops = 1 tsp
    1 fl oz = 6 tsp = 2 Tbs = 29.573 mL
    1 cup = 8 fl oz = 250 mL

Dry Measures
    5 g = 1 tsp dried, powdered herb
    10 g = 2 tsp dried, powdered herb
    3 tsp = 1 Tbs = approx. 1/2 oz dried powdered herb

INDEX